DASH
Diet Cookbook
For Families

2 Books in 1 | Dr. Cole's Funny
Meal Plan | Budget Friendly Low
Sodium Recipes for Whole Family |
An Easy Way to Take Care of your
Kids

By Janeth Cole

ISBN: 978-1-80301-498-2 (Paperback)

ISBN: 978-1-80301-499-9 (Hardcover)

Table of Contents

1st Book

DASH Diet Cookbook for Women

2nd Book

DASH Diet Cookbook On a Budget

DASH
Diet Cookbook
For Women

Simple Dr. Cole's Meal Plan |
Delicious and Affordable Low
Sodium Recipes to Weight Loss and
Lower Blood Pressure

By Janeth Cole

Chapter 1 -   Introduction

The Dietary Approaches to Stop Hypertension better known as the DASH diet is more than a fad or a trend, it can really make a difference in your health and your appearance. In contrast to other diets, the DASH diet emerged from a group of specialists in 1997 with the goal of reducing high blood pressure. Later, other benefits were found, including the prevention of type II diabetes and help during menopause.

In a research conducted by Valentino, Giovanna, Tagle, Rodrigo, & Acevedo, Mónica (2014) mention the benefits of DASH diet during menopause as a treatment that mitigates the effects caused by the decrease in estrogen production.

Dash Diet Manifesto

The central manifesto of the DASH diet is to reduce dietary sodium to below 2.3 g in regular DASH and 1.5 g in low sodium DASH (equivalent to 3.8 g of salt); increasing consumption of foods rich in potassium, calcium, fiber and magnesium.

In simple terms, it consists of reducing the intake of salt, fats and sugars as much as possible.

What foods can I eat on the DASH diet?

The first thing you should consider is the reduction or elimination of fatty foods, sugary or processed products. You should increase your intake of fresh fruits and vegetables, nuts and seeds, whole grains and dried fruits, fish and lean meat, low-fat or fat-free dairy products. For cooking or frying your food you can opt for olive, coconut or soybean oil.

It also encourages you to stay hydrated by drinking 2 liters of water daily, which also allows you to eliminate excess sodium. Use low-fat cooking techniques such as grilling, broiling, roasting, baking, microwaving or steaming cooking.

Benefits to women

There are many benefits of the DASH diet for all women no matter what age or stage of life you are in, for example: it is your ally during menopause and pre-menopause, helps you lose weight, controls high blood pressure, prevents type II diabetes, reduces the risk of heart disease, controls and improves cholesterol levels, prevents the development of annoying kidney stones. Discover that eating smart is the best way to a fit and healthy body.

Valentino, Giovanna, Tagle, Rodrigo, & Acevedo, Mónica. (2014). Dieta DASH y menopausia: Más allá de los beneficios en hipertensión arterial. *Revista chilena de cardiología*, 33(3), 215-222. https://dx.doi.org/10.4067/S0718-85602014000300008

Chapter 2 -   Breakfast Recipes

1) Cheesy Red Omelette

Preparation Time: 5 minutes

Cooking Time: 10 minutes

Servings: 4

Nutrition: Calories: 191 Fat: 15g Carbs: 6g Protein: 9g

Ingredients:

- 2 tablespoons olive oil
- 1 medium onion, chopped
- 1 teaspoon garlic, minced
- 2 medium tomatoes, chopped
- 6 large eggs
- ½ cup half and half
- ½ cup feta cheese, crumbled
- ¼ cup dill weed
- Ground black pepper as needed

Directions:

- ❖ Pre-heat your oven to a temperature of 400 degrees Fahrenheit. Take a large sized ovenproof pan and heat up your olive oil over medium-high heat. Toss in the onion, garlic, tomatoes and stir fry them for 4 minutes.
- ❖ While they are being cooked, take a bowl and beat together your eggs, half and half cream and season the mix with some pepper.
- ❖ Pour the mixture into the pan with your vegetables and top it with crumbled feta cheese and dill weed. Cover it with the lid and let it cook for 3 minutes.
- ❖ Place the pan inside your oven and let it bake for 10 minutes. Serve hot.

2) Apple Warm Oatmeal

Preparation Time: 10 minutes

Cooking Time: 4 minutes

Servings: 3

Nutrition: calories 200, fat 1g, carbs 12g, protein 10g

Ingredients:

- 3 cups water
- 1 cup steel cut oats
- 1 apple, cored and chopped
- 1 tablespoon cinnamon powder

Directions:

- ❖ In your instant pot, mix water with oats, cinnamon and apple, stir, cover and Cooking Time: on High for 4 minutes.
- ❖ Stir again, divide into bowls and serve for breakfast.
- ❖ Enjoy!

3) Golden Coco Mix

Preparation Time: 15 minutes

Cooking Time: 0 minutes

Servings: 6

Nutrition: Calories: 259 Fat: 13g Carbs: 5g Protein: 16g

Ingredients:

- Powdered erythritol as needed
- 1 ½ cups almond milk, unsweetened
- 2 tablespoons vanilla protein powder
- 3 tablespoons Golden Flaxseed meal
- 2 tablespoons coconut flour

Directions:

- ❖ Take a bowl and mix in flaxseed meal, protein powder, coconut flour and mix well. Add mix to saucepan (placed over medium heat).
- ❖ Add almond milk and stir, let the mixture thicken. Add your desired amount of sweetener and serve. Enjoy!

4) Delicious Agave Rice

Preparation Time: 10 minutes

Cooking Time: 7 minutes

Servings: 4

Nutrition: calories 192, fat 1g, carbs 20g, protein 4g

Ingredients:

- 1 cup Arborio rice
- 2 cups almond milk
- 1 cup coconut milk
- 1/3 cup agave nectar
- 2 teaspoons vanilla extract
- ¼ cup coconut flakes, toasted

Directions:

- ❖ Set your instant pot on simmer mode, add almond and coconut milk and bring to a boil.
- ❖ Add agave nectar and rice, stir, cover and Cooking Time: on High for 5 minutes.
- ❖ Add vanilla and coconut, stir, divide into bowls and serve warm.
- ❖ Enjoy!

5) Italian Feta Breakfast Eggs

Preparation Time: 5 minutes

Cooking Time: 15 minutes

Servings: 12

Nutrition: Calories: 106 Fat: 8g Carbs: 2g Protein: 7g

Ingredients:

- 2 tablespoons of unsalted butter (replace with canola oil for full effect)
- ½ cup of chopped up scallions
- 1 cup of crumbled feta cheese
- 8 large sized eggs
- 2/3 cup of milk
- ½ teaspoon of dried Italian seasoning
- Freshly ground black pepper as needed
- Cooking oil spray

Directions:

- ❖ Pre-heat your oven to 400 degrees Fahrenheit. Take a 3-4 ounce muffin pan and grease with cooking oil. Take a non-stick pan and place it over medium heat.
- ❖ Add butter and allow the butter to melt. Add half of the scallions and stir fry. Keep them to the side. Take a medium-sized bowl and add eggs, Italian seasoning and milk and whisk well.
- ❖ Add the stir fried scallions and feta cheese and mix. Season with pepper. Pour the mix into the muffin tin. Transfer the muffin tin to your oven and bake for 15 minutes. Serve with a sprinkle of scallions.

6) *Cinnamon Pumpkin Oatmeal with Vanilla Flavour*

Preparation Time: 10 minutes

Cooking Time: 3 minutes

Servings: 6

Nutrition: calories 173, fat 1g, carbs 20g, protein 6g

Ingredients:

- 4 and ½ cups water
- 1 and ½ cups steel cut oats
- 2 teaspoons cinnamon powder
- 1 teaspoon vanilla extract
- 1 teaspoon allspice
- 1 and ½ cup pumpkin puree
- ¼ cup pecans, chopped

Directions:

- ❖ In your instant pot, mix water with oats, cinnamon, vanilla allspice and pumpkin puree, stir, cover and Cooking Time: on High for 3 minutes.
- ❖ Divide into bowls, stir again, cool down and serve with pecans on top.
- ❖ Enjoy!

7) *Button Mushroom Omelette*

Preparation Time: 5 minutes

Cooking Time: 15 minutes

Servings: 4

Nutrition: Calories: 189 Fat: 13g Carbs: 6g Protein: 12g

Ingredients:

- 2 tablespoons of butter (replace with canola oil for full effect)
- 1 chopped up medium-sized onion
- 2 minced cloves of garlic
- 1 cup of coarsely chopped baby rocket tomato
- 1 cup of sliced button mushrooms
- 6 large pieces of eggs
- ½ cup of skim milk
- 1 teaspoon of dried rosemary
- Ground black pepper as needed

Directions:

- ❖ Pre-heat your oven to 400 degrees Fahrenheit. Take a large oven-proof pan and place it over medium-heat. Heat up some oil.
- ❖ Stir fry your garlic, onion for about 2 minutes. Add the mushroom, rosemary and rockets and cook for 3 minutes. Take a medium-sized bowl and beat your eggs alongside the milk.
- ❖ Season it with some pepper. Pour the egg mixture into your pan with the vegetables and sprinkle some Parmesan.
- ❖ Reduce the heat to low and cover with the lid. Let it cook for 3 minutes. Transfer the pan into your oven and bake for 10 minutes until fully settled.
- ❖ Reduce the heat to low and cover with your lid. Let it cook for 3 minutes. Transfer the pan into your oven and then bake for another 10 minutes. Serve hot.

8) *Easy Tofu Bowl*

Preparation Time: 10 minutes

Cooking Time: 10 minutes

Servings: 4

Nutrition: calories 172, fat 7g, carbs 20g, protein 6g

Ingredients:

- 1 pound extra firm tofu, cubed
- 1 cup sweet potato, chopped
- 3 garlic cloves, minced
- 2 tablespoons sesame seeds
- 1 yellow onion, chopped
- 2 teaspoons sesame seed oil
- 1 carrot, chopped
- 1 tablespoon tamari
- 1 tablespoon rice vinegar
- 2 cups snow peas, halved
- 1/3 cup veggie stock
- 2 tablespoons red pepper sauce
- 2 tablespoons scallions, chopped
- 2 tablespoons tahini paste

Directions:

- ❖ Set your instant pot on sauté mode, add oil, heat it up, add sweet potato, onion and carrots, stir and Cooking Time: for 2 minutes.
- ❖ Add garlic, half of the sesame seeds, tofu, vinegar, tamari and stock, stir and Cooking Time: for 2 minutes more.
- ❖ Cover pot and Cooking Time: on High for 3 minutes more.
- ❖ Add peas, the rest of the sesame seeds, green onions, tahini paste and pepper sauce, stir, cover and Cooking Time: on Low for 1 minutes more.
- ❖ Divide into bowls and serve for breakfast.
- ❖ Enjoy!

9) *Canned Beans and Tomato Breads*

Preparation Time: 5 minutes

Cooking Time: 15 minutes

Servings: 4

Nutrition: Calories 382 Fat: 1.8g Carbs: 66g Protein: 28.5g

Ingredients:

- 1 ½ tbsp olive oil
- 1 tomato, cubed
- 1 garlic clove, minced
- 1 red onion, chopped
- ¼ cup parsley, chopped
- 15 oz. canned fava beans, drained and rinsed
- ¼ cup lemon juice
- Black pepper to the taste
- 4 whole-wheat pita bread pockets

Directions:

- ❖ Heat a pan with the oil over medium heat, add the onion, stir, and sauté for 5 minutes. Add the rest of the ingredients, stir, and cook for 10 minutes more
- ❖ Stuff the pita pockets with this mix and serve for breakfast.

10) Black Olives and Feta Bread

Preparation Time: 1 hour and 40 minutes

Cooking Time: 30 minutes

Servings: 10

Nutrition: Calories 251 Fat: 7.3g Carbs: 39.7g Protein: 6.7g

Ingredients:

- 4 cups whole-wheat flour
- 3 tbsps. oregano, chopped
- 2 tsps. dry yeast
- ¼ cup olive oil
- 1 ½ cups black olives, pitted and sliced
- 1 cup of water
- ½ cup feta cheese, crumbled

Directions:

- ❖ In a bowl, mix the flour with the water, the yeast, and the oil. Stir and knead your dough very well. Put the dough in a bowl, cover with plastic wrap, and keep in a warm place for 1 hour.
- ❖ Divide the dough into 2 bowls and stretch each ball well. Add the rest of the ingredients to each ball and tuck them inside. Knead the dough well again.
- ❖ Flatten the balls a bit and leave them aside for 40 minutes more. Transfer the balls to a baking sheet lined with parchment paper, make a small slit in each, and bake at 425F for 30 minutes.
- ❖ Serve the bread as a Mediterranean breakfast.

11) Lentils and Mushroom Burgers

Preparation Time: 10 minutes

Cooking Time: 30 minutes

Servings: 4

Nutrition: calories 140, fat 3g, carbs 14g, protein 13g

Ingredients:

- 1 cup mushrooms, chopped
- 2 teaspoons ginger, grated
- 1 cup yellow onion, chopped
- 1 cup red lentils
- 1 sweet potato, chopped
- 2 and ½ cups veggie stock
- ¼ cup hemp seeds
- ¼ cup parsley, chopped
- 1 tablespoon curry powder
- ¼ cup cilantro, chopped
- 1 cup quick oats
- 4 tablespoons rice flour

Direction:

- ❖ Set your instant pot on sauté mode, add onion, mushrooms and ginger, stir and sauté for 2 minutes.
- ❖ Add lentils, stock and sweet potatoes, stir, cover and Cooking Time: on High for 6 minutes.
- ❖ Leave this mixture aside to cool down, mash using a potato masher, add parsley, hemp, curry powder, cilantro, oats and rice flour and stir well.
- ❖ Shape 8 patties out of this mix, arrange them all on a lined baking sheet, introduce in the oven at 375 degrees F and bake for 10 minutes on each side.
- ❖ Divide between plates and serve for breakfast.
- ❖ Enjoy!

12) Cheesy Baked Potato

Preparation Time: 10 minutes

Cooking Time: 1 hour and 10 minutes

Servings: 8

Nutrition: Calories 476 Fat: 16.8g Carbs: 68.8g Protein: 13.9g

Ingredients:

- 2 pounds sweet potatoes, peeled and cubed
- ¼ cup olive oil + a drizzle
- 7 oz. feta cheese, crumbled
- 1 yellow onion, chopped
- 2 eggs, whisked
- ¼ cup almond milk
- 1 tbsp. herbs de Provence
- A pinch of black pepper
- 6 phyllo sheets
- 1 tbsp. parmesan, grated

Directions:

- ❖ In a bowl, combine the potatoes with half of the oil, and pepper, toss, spread on a baking sheet lined with parchment paper, and roast at 400F for 25 minutes.
- ❖ Meanwhile, heat a pan with half of the remaining oil over medium heat, add the onion, and sauté for 5 minutes.
- ❖ In a bowl, combine the eggs with the milk, feta, herbs, pepper, onion, sweet potatoes, and the rest of the oil and toss.
- ❖ Arrange the phyllo sheets in a tart pan and brush them with a drizzle of oil. Add the sweet potato mix and spread it well into the pan.
- ❖ Sprinkle the parmesan on top and bake covered with tin foil at 350F for 20 minutes. Remove the tin foil, bake the tart for 20 minutes more, cool it down, slice, and serve for breakfast.

13) Breakfast Walnuts Quinoa

Preparation Time: 5 minutes

Cooking Time: 0 minutes

Servings: 4

Nutrition: Calories 284 Fat: 14.3g Carbs: 15.4g Protein: 4.4g

Ingredients:

- 2 cups almond milk
- 2 cups quinoa, already cooked
- ½ tsp cinnamon powder
- 1 tbsp. honey
- 1 cup blueberries
- ¼ cup walnuts, chopped

Directions:

- ❖ In a bowl, mix the quinoa with the milk and the rest of the ingredients, toss, divide into smaller bowls and serve for breakfast

14) Vegetables Wraps with Soy Sauce

Preparation Time: 10 minutes

Cooking Time: 15 minutes

Servings: 6

Nutrition: calories 100, fat 2g, carbs 9g, protein 3g

Ingredients:

- 1 tablespoon olive oil
- 1 cup mushrooms, chopped
- 1 and ½ cups cabbage, chopped
- ½ cup carrots, grated
- 1 and ½ cups water
- 2 tablespoons soy sauce
- 1 teaspoon ginger, grated
- 1 tablespoon rice wine vinegar
- 1 teaspoon sesame oil
- 12 vegan dumpling wrappers

Directions:

- ❖ Set your instant pot on sauté mode, add olive oil, heat it up, add mushrooms, stir and Cooking Time: for 2 minutes.
- ❖ Add carrot, cabbage, soy sauce and vinegar, stir and Cooking Time: for 3 minutes more.
- ❖ Add sesame oil and ginger, stir and transfer everything to a bowl.
- ❖ Arrange all wrappers on a working surface, divide veggie mix, wrap them and seal with some water.
- ❖ Add the water to your instant pot, add steamer basket, add dumplings inside, cover pot and Cooking Time: on High for 7 minutes.
- ❖ Divide between plates and serve for breakfast.
- ❖ Enjoy!

15) Brown Rice and Chickpeas Breakfast Bowl

Preparation Time: Breakfast Rice Bowl

Cooking Time: 30 minutes

Servings: 4

Nutrition: calories 292, fat 4g, carbs 9g, protein 10g

Ingredients:

- 1 tablespoon olive oil
- 2 tablespoons chana masala
- 1 red onion, chopped
- 1 tablespoon ginger, grated
- 1 tablespoon garlic, minced
- 1 cup chickpeas
- 3 cups water
- A pinch of black pepper
- 14 ounces tomatoes, chopped
- 1 and ½ cups brown rice

Directions:

- ❖ Set your instant pot on sauté mode, add the oil, heat it up, add onion, stir and Cooking Time: for 7 minutes.
- ❖ Add pepper, chana masala, ginger and garlic, stir and Cooking Time: for 1
- ❖ minute more.
- ❖ Add tomatoes, chickpeas, rice and water, stir, cover and Cooking Time: on High for 20 minutes.
- ❖ Stir one more time, divide into bowls and serve for breakfast.
- ❖ Enjoy!

16) Sauté Vegan Millet

Preparation Time: 10 minutes

Cooking Time: 16 minutes

Servings: 4

Nutrition: calories 172, fat 3g, carbs 19g, protein 5g

Ingredients:

- 1 cup millet
- ½ cup oyster mushrooms, chopped
- 2 garlic cloves, minced
- ½ cup green lentils
- ½ cup bok choy, chopped
- 2 and ¼ cups veggie stock
- 1 cup yellow onion, chopped
- 1 cup asparagus, chopped
- 1 tablespoon lemon juice
- ¼ cup parsley and chives, chopped

Directions:

- ❖ Set your instant pot on sauté mode, heat it up, add garlic, onion and mushrooms, stir and Cooking Time: for 2 minutes.
- ❖ Add lentils and millet, stir and Cooking Time: for a few seconds more.
- ❖ Add stock, stir, cover and Cooking Time: on High for 10 minutes.
- ❖ Add asparagus and bok choy, stir, cover and leave everything aside for 3 minutes.
- ❖ Add parsley and chives and lemon juice, stir, divide into bowls and serve for breakfast.
- ❖ Enjoy!

17) Black Navel Salad

Preparation Time: 5 minutes

Cooking Time: 0 minutes

Servings: 4

Nutrition: Calories 97 Fat: 9.1g Carbs: 3.7g Protein: 1.9g

Ingredients:

- 1 tbsp. balsamic vinegar
- 2 garlic cloves, minced
- 1 tsp. Dijon mustard
- 2 tbsps. olive oil
- 1 tbsp. lemon juice
- Black pepper to taste
- ½ cup black olives, pitted and chopped
- 1 tbsp. parsley, chopped
- 7 cups baby spinach
- 2 endives, shredded
- 3 medium navel oranges, peeled and cut into segments
- 2 bulbs fennel, shredded

Directions:

- ❖ In a salad bowl, combine the spinach with the endives, oranges, fennel, and the rest of the ingredients, toss and serve for breakfast.

18) Almond Pearls Pudding

Preparation Time: 10 minutes

Cooking Time: 8 minutes

Servings: 4

Nutrition: calories 187, fat 3g, fiber 1g, carbs 18g, protein 3g

Ingredients:

- 1/3 cup tapioca pearls
- ½ cup water
- 1 and ¼ cups almond milk
- ½ cup stevia
- Zest from ½ lemon, grated

Directions:

- ❖ In a heatproof bowl, mix tapioca with almond milk, stevia and lemon zest and stir well.
- ❖ Add the water to your instant pot, add steamer basket, and heatproof bowl inside, cover and Cooking Time: on High for 8 minutes.
- ❖ Stir your pudding and serve for breakfast.
- ❖ Enjoy!

19) Awesome Brakfast Muesli

Preparation Time: 15 minutes

Cooking Time: 20 minutes

Servings: 8

Nutrition: Calories 250 Fat: 10g Carbs: 36g Protein: 7g

Ingredients:

- 3 ½ cups rolled oats
- ½ cup wheat bran
- ½ tsp ground cinnamon
- ½ cup sliced almonds
- ¼ cup raw pecans, coarsely chopped
- ¼ cup raw pepitas (shelled pumpkin seeds)
- ½ cup unsweetened coconut flakes
- ¼ cup dried apricots, coarsely chopped
- ¼ cup dried cherries

Directions:

- ❖ Take a medium bowl and combine the oats, wheat bran and cinnamon. Stir well. Place the mixture onto a baking sheet.
- ❖ Next place the almonds, pecans, and pepitas onto another baking sheet and toss. Pop both trays into the oven and heat to 350°F. Bake for 10-12 minutes. Remove from the oven and pop to one side.
- ❖ Leave the nuts to cool but take the one with the oats, sprinkle with the coconut, and pop back into the oven for 5 minutes more. Remove and leave to cool.
- ❖ Find a large bowl and combine the contents of both trays then stir well to combine. Throw in the apricots and cherries and stir well. Pop into an airtight container until required.

20) Delicious Kamut Salad with Walnuts

Preparation Time: 10 minutes

Cooking Time: 15 minutes

Servings: 6

Nutrition: calories 125, fat 6g, fiber 2g, carbs 4g, protein 3g

Ingredients:

- 2 cups water
- 1 cup kamut grains, soaked for 12 hours, drained and mixed with some lemon juice
- 1 teaspoon sunflower oil
- 4 ounces arugula
- 2 blood oranges, peeled and cut into medium segments
- 1 tablespoon olive oil
- 3 ounces walnuts, chopped

Directions:

- ❖ In your instant pot, mix kamut grains with sunflower oil and the water, stir, cover and Cooking Time: on High for 15 minutes.
- ❖ Drain kamut, transfer to a bowl, add a
- ❖ pinch of salt, arugula, orange segments, oil and walnuts, toss well and serve for breakfast.
- ❖ Enjoy!

Chapter 3 -   Rice & Grain and Pasta Recipes

21) Pasta with Delicious Spanish Salsa

Preparation Time: 15 minutes

Cooking Time:

Servings: 2

Nutrition: Carbs: 69g Protein: 12.7g Fats: 2.3g Calories: 364

Ingredients:
- Spaghetti : 160g
- Red onion: ½ roughly chopped
- Green pepper: 1 chopped
- Cherry tomatoes:250g
- Tabasco: a good dash
- Garlic: ½ clove
- Vinegar: 1 tbsp
- Basi l a small bunch

Directions:
- ❖ Cooking Time: pasta as per packet instructions
- ❖ In the meanwhile, take a blender and add tomatoes, garlic, onion, and pepper, and blend
- ❖ Add in Tabasco and vinegar and combine well
- ❖ Add the sauce to the paste
- ❖ Top with basil and serve

22) Penne with Zucchini and Wine

Preparation Time: 15 minutes

Cooking Time: 30 minutes

Servings: 6

Nutrition: Calories: 340 Fat: 6.2g Protein: 8.0g Carbs: 66.8g

Ingredients:
- 1 large zucchini, diced
- 1 large butternut squash, peeled and diced
- 1 large yellow onion, chopped
- 2 tablespoons extra-virgin olive oil
- 1 teaspoon paprika
- ½ teaspoon garlic powder
- ½ teaspoon freshly ground black pepper
- 1 pound (454 g) whole-grain penne
- ½ cup dry white wine
- 2 tablespoons grated Parmesan cheese

Directions:
- ❖ Preheat the oven to 400°F (205°C). Line a baking sheet with aluminum foil. Combine the zucchini, butternut squash, and onion in a large bowl.
- ❖ Drizzle with olive oil and sprinkle with paprika, garlic powder, and ground black pepper. Toss to coat well.
- ❖ Spread the vegetables in the single layer on the baking sheet, then roast in the preheated oven for 25 minutes or until the vegetables are tender.
- ❖ Meanwhile, bring a pot of water to a boil, then add the penne and cook for 14 minutes or until al dente. Drain the penne through a colander.
- ❖ Transfer ½ cup of roasted vegetables in a food processor, then pour in the dry white wine. Pulse until smooth.
- ❖ Pour the puréed vegetables in a nonstick skillet and cook with penne over medium-high heat for a few minutes to heat through.
- ❖ Transfer the penne with the purée on a large serving plate, then spread the remaining roasted vegetables and Parmesan on top before serving.

23) Gochujang and Carrot Spaghetti with Coriander

Preparation Time: 45 minutes

Cooking Time:

Servings: 2

Nutrition: Carbs: 52.5g Protein: 10.9g Fats: 15.5g Calories: 404

Ingredients:
- Spaghetti: 2 cups
- Olive oil: 2 tbsp
- Cauliflower: 2 cups cut in big florets
- Gochujang: 2 tbsp
- Rice vinegar: 1 tbsp
- Sliced red pepper: 1 cup sliced
- Carrot: 2 sliced
- Pepper: as per your taste
- Coriander: 1⁄2 cup chopped

Directions:
- ❖ Cooking Time: spaghetti as per packet instructions
- ❖ Preheat the oven 200C
- ❖ Add cauliflowers to the baking sheet and sprinkle seasoning and brush with olive oil
- ❖ Roast for 25 minutes till it turns golden and soft
- ❖ Remove from oven and brush with gochujang and Cooking Time: in the oven again for 10 minutes
- ❖ Add to the bowl and mix with carrots and red bell pepper
- ❖ Season with coriander, and pepper and pour vinegar from top
- ❖ Spread spaghetti on the serving tray and top with the cauliflower

24) Spinach Cheesy Pasta

Preparation Time: 15 minutes

Cooking Time: 14-16 minutes

Servings: 4

Nutrition: Calories: 262 Fat: 4.0g Protein: 15.0g Carbs: 51.0g

Ingredients:

- 8 ounces (227 g) uncooked penne
- 1 tablespoon extra-virgin olive oil
- 2 garlic cloves, minced
- ¼ teaspoon crushed red pepper
- 2 cups chopped fresh flat-leaf parsley, including stems
- 5 cups loosely packed baby spinach
- ¼ teaspoon ground nutmeg
- ¼ teaspoon freshly ground black pepper
- 1/3 cup Castelvetrano olives, pitted and sliced
- 1/3 cup grated Parmesan cheese

Directions:

- ❖ In a large stockpot of salted water, cook the pasta for about 8 to 10 minutes. Drain the pasta and reserve ¼ cup of the cooking liquid.
- ❖ Meanwhile, heat the olive oil in a large skillet over medium heat. Add the garlic and red pepper and cook for 30 seconds, stirring constantly.
- ❖ Add the parsley and cook for 1 minute, stirring constantly. Add the spinach, nutmeg and pepper, and cook for 3 minutes, stirring occasionally, or until the spinach is wilted.
- ❖ Add the cooked pasta and the reserved ¼ cup cooking liquid to the skillet. Stir in the olives and cook for about 2 minutes, or until most of the pasta water has been absorbed.
- ❖ Remove from the heat and stir in the cheese before serving.

25) Chickpeas Tomato Pasta with Tamari

Preparation Time: 30 minutes

Cooking Time:

Servings: 2

Nutrition: Carbs: 54g Protein: 14.6g Fats: 18g Calories: 442

Ingredients:

- Pasta: 1 cup cooked
- Chickpeas: 1 cup rinsed and drained well
- Onion: 1 cup finely diced
- Tomato: 2 cups diced
- Lemon juice: 2 tbsp
- Kale: 1 cup
- Olive oil: 2 tbsp
- Tamari: 1 tbsp
- Coriander: 2 tbsp chopped
- Garlic: 1 clove crushed

Directions:

- ❖ Cooking Time: pasta as per packet instructions
- ❖ Add garlic, lemon juice, tamari, and olive oil in a bowl and whisk
- ❖ Take a serving bowl and combine kale, pasta, chickpeas, onion, tomatoes, and the sauce you made
- ❖ Add coriander from the top and serve

26) Italian Tricolor Pasta

Preparation Time: 5 minutes

Cooking Time: 25 minutes

Servings: 6

Nutrition: Calories: 147 Fat: 3.0g Protein: 16.0g Carbs: 17.0g

Ingredients:

- 8 ounces (227 g) uncooked small pasta, like orecchiette (little ears) or farfalle (bow ties)
- 1½ pounds (680 g) fresh asparagus, ends trimmed and stalks chopped into 1-inch pieces
- 1½ cups grape tomatoes, halved
- 2 tablespoons extra-virgin olive oil
- ¼ teaspoon freshly ground black pepper
- 2 cups fresh Mozzarella, drained and cut into bite-size pieces (about 8 ounces / 227 g)
- 1/3 cup torn fresh basil leaves
- 2 tablespoons balsamic vinegar

Directions:

- ❖ Preheat the oven to 400°F (205°C). In a large stockpot of salted water, cook the pasta for about 8 to 10 minutes. Drain and reserve about ¼ cup of the cooking liquid.
- ❖ Meanwhile, in a large bowl, toss together the asparagus, tomatoes, oil and pepper. Spread the mixture onto a large, rimmed baking sheet and bake in the oven for 15 minutes, stirring twice during cooking.
- ❖ Remove the vegetables from the oven and add the cooked pasta to the baking sheet. Mix with a few tablespoons of cooking liquid to help the sauce become smoother and the saucy vegetables stick to the pasta.
- ❖ Gently mix in the Mozzarella and basil. Drizzle with the balsamic vinegar. Serve from the baking sheet or pour the pasta into a large bowl.

27) *Fusilli with Juicy Cauliflowers*

Preparation Time: 20 minutes

Cooking Time:

Servings: 2

Nutrition: Carbs: 21.6g Protein: 4.85g Fats: 7.9g Calories: 172

Ingredients:
- Fusilli: 1 cup cooked
- Cauliflower: 1 cup roughly chopped
- Garlic: 2 cloves thinly sliced
- Olive oil: 1 tbsp
- Chili flakes: 1 tsp
- Pepper: as per your taste
- Lemon: 1 juice and zest

Directions:
- Cooking Time: the pasta as per the packet instruction
- Add cauliflower when the pasta is about to be done
- Drain but keep one cup of the water
- Take a large pan and heat oil
- Add in garlic and Cooking Time: for two minutes
- Add in chili and Cooking Time: for a minutes
- Add pasta, lemon juice and zest, pepper, and cauliflower with the pasta water
- Mix everything well and serve

28) *Shrimp Fettuccine with Black Pepper*

Preparation Time: 15 minutes

Cooking Time: 15 minutes

Servings: 4-6

Nutrition: Calories: 615 Fat: 17.0g Protein: 33.0g Carbs: 89.0g

Ingredients:
- 8 ounces (227 g) fettuccine pasta
- ¼ cup extra-virgin olive oil
- 3 tablespoons garlic, minced
- 1 pound (454 g) large shrimp, peeled and deveined
- 1/3 cup lemon juice
- 1 tablespoon lemon zest
- ½ teaspoon freshly ground black pepper

Directions:
- Bring a large pot of water to a boil. Add the fettuccine and cook for 8 minutes. Reserve ½ cup of the cooking liquid and drain the pasta.
- In a large saucepan over medium heat, heat the olive oil. Add the garlic and sauté for 1 minute.
- Add the shrimp to the saucepan and cook each side for 3 minutes. Remove the shrimp from the pan and set aside.
- Add the remaining ingredients to the saucepan. Stir in the cooking liquid. Add the pasta and toss together to evenly coat the pasta.
- Transfer the pasta to a serving dish and serve topped with the cooked shrimp.

29) *Spiced Kidney Pasta with Cilantro*

Preparation Time: 30 minutes

Cooking Time:

Servings: 4

Nutrition: Carbs: 41.98g Protein: 9.3g Fats: 8.4g Calories: 274

Ingredients:
- Pasta: 2 cups (after cooking
- Onion: 1 chopped
- Garlic: 1 ½ tsp minced
- Cumin: 1 tsp
- Frozen corn: 1 cup
- Cayenne pepper: ¼ tsp
- Kidney beans: 1 cup drained and rinsed
- Fresh cilantro: 2 tsp
- Lemon juice: 3 tbsp
- Cooking oil: 2 tbsp

Directions:
- Cooking Time: pasta as per packet instructions
- Take a saucepan and heat oil in it
- Add garlic and onion to it and make them tender
- Add cayenne pepper, and cumin
- Now add corns and beans and mix well
- Cover and Cooking Time: for 5 minutes
- Add in pasta and stir and remove from heat after 5 minutes
- Pour lemon juice on top
- Garnish with cilantro and serve

30) *Classic Grandma's Pasta*

Preparation Time: 15 minutes

Cooking Time: 25 minutes

Servings: 4

Nutrition: Calories 500 Fat 18.3 g Carbohydrates 69.7 g Protein 16.2 g

Ingredients:
- 1 pack of 16 angel hair pasta
- 1/4 cup of olive oil
- 1/2 onion, minced
- 4 cloves of chopped garlic
- 2 cups of Roma tomatoes, diced
- 2 tablespoons balsamic vinegar
- 1 low-sodium chicken broth
- ground red pepper
- freshly ground black pepper to taste
- 1/4 cup grated Parmesan cheese
- 2 tablespoons chopped fresh basil

Directions:
- Bring a large pot of water to a boil. Add pasta and cook for 8 minutes or until al dente; drain.
- Pour the olive oil in a large deep pan over high heat. Fry onions and garlic until light brown. Lower the heat to medium and add tomatoes, vinegar, and chicken stock; simmer for about 8 minutes.
- Stir in the red pepper, black pepper, basil, and cooked pasta and mix well with the sauce. Simmer for about 5 minutes and serve garnished with grated cheese.

31) Red Lentils Spaghetti with Herbs

Preparation Time: :45 minutes

Cooking Time:

Servings: 2

Nutrition: Carbs: 33.33g Protein: 13.3g Fats: 15.1g Calories: 335.2

Ingredients:

- Spaghetti: 1 cup cooked
- Red lentils: 1 cup
- Potato: 1 cup diced
- Crushed tomatoes: 2 cups
- Onion: 1 diced
- Ginger: 1 tbsp paste
- Garlic: 1 tbsp paste
- Vegetable oil: 2 tbsp
- Water: 4 cups
- Italian herb seasoning: 1 tbsp
- Pepper: as per your taste

Directions:

- ❖ Cooking Time: spaghetti as per packet instructions
- ❖ Take a large saucepan and heat oil on a medium flame
- ❖ Add onion and ginger and garlic paste and sauté for 3-4 minutes
- ❖ Pour water and bring to boil
- ❖ Add lentils, potatoes and bring to boil
- ❖ Lower the heat to medium and Cooking Time: for 20 minutes with partial cover
- ❖ Now add crushed tomatoes to the lentils along with Italian herb seasoning and pepper
- ❖ Cooking Time: on low flame for 15 minutes
- ❖ Add the mixture to the high-speed blender to make a puree
- ❖ Add in spaghetti pasta and mix well
- ❖ Add pepper to augment the taste

32) Spicy Shrimp Pasta with Bay Scallops

Preparation Time: 15 minutes

Cooking Time: 55 minutes

Servings: 8

Nutrition: Calories 335 Fat 8.9 g Carbs 46.3 g Protein 18.7 g

Ingredients:

- 4 tablespoons olive oil, divided
- 6 cloves of garlic, crushed
- 3 cups peeled whole tomatoes with liquid, chopped
- 1 teaspoon crushed red pepper flakes
- 1 packet of linguine pasta
- 8 grams of small shrimp, peeled
- 8 grams of bay scallops
- 1 tablespoon of chopped fresh parsley

Directions:

- ❖ Heat 2 tablespoons of olive oil and sauté garlic over medium heat. When the garlic starts to sizzle, pour in the tomatoes.
- ❖ Season with red pepper. Bring to boil. Reduce the heat and simmer for 30 minutes, stirring occasionally.
- ❖ Meanwhile, boil a large pan with lightly salted water. Cook pasta for about 8 to 10 minutes or until al dente; drain.
- ❖ Heat the remaining 2 tablespoons of olive oil in a large frying pan over high heat. Add shrimps and scallops. Cook for about 2 minutes stirring regularly, or until the shrimp turn pink.
- ❖ Add the shrimp and scallops to the tomato mixture and stir in the parsley. Bake for 3 to 4 minutes or until the sauce starts to bubble. Serve the sauce on the pasta.

33) Italian Pasta e Fagioli

Preparation Time: 30 minutes

Cooking Time:

Servings: 2

Nutrition: Carbs: 39.2g Protein: 11.3g Fats: 8.2g Calories: 272

Ingredients:

- Pasta: 1 cup (after cooking
- Olive oil: 1 tbsp
- Beans: 1 cup can rinsed and drained
- Garlic: 2 cloves minced
- Tomato paste: ¼ cup
- Red onion: 1 small diced
- Red chili flakes: 1 tsp
- Black pepper: ½ tsp
- Parsley: ½ cup

Directions:

- ❖ Cooking Time: pasta as per packet instructions
- ❖ Take a saucepan and heat oil in it
- ❖ Add minced garlic and onion to it and
- ❖ make them tender
- ❖ Add beans, pepper, tomato paste, and red chili flakes and mix well
- ❖ Add cooked pasta and stir
- ❖ Lower the heat and cover and Cooking Time: for 5 minutes and then remove from heat
- ❖ Sprinkle parsley on top and serve

34) Penne with Vodka Cream

Preparation Time: 15 minutes

Cooking Time: 25 minutes

Servings: 8

Nutrition: Calories 435 Fat 18.4 g Carbs 52.7 g Protein 13.3 g

Ingredients:
- 1-pound uncooked penne
- 1/4 cup extra virgin olive oil
- 4 cloves finely chopped garlic
- 1/2 teaspoon crushed red pepper flakes
- 1 can of crushed tomatoes
- 2 tablespoons of vodka
- 1/2 cup thick whipped cream
- 1/4 cup chopped fresh parsley
- 2 (3.5 ounces) sweet Italian sausage links

Directions:
- ❖ Bring a large pan of water to a boil. Put the pasta and cook for 8 to 10 minutes or until al dente; drain.
- ❖ Heat the oil in a large frying pan over medium heat. Remove the casing from the sausage and add it to the pan.
- ❖ Cook by browning the meat, add garlic and red pepper and cook, stirring until the garlic is golden brown. Add tomatoes and boil. Lower the heat and simmer for 15 minutes.
- ❖ Add vodka and cream and bring to a boil. Reduce the heat and add the pasta, mix for 1 minute. Stir in the fresh parsley and serve!

35) Macaroni with Cherry and Peas

Preparation Time: 40 minutes

Cooking Time:

Servings: 2

Nutrition: Carbs: 37.5g Protein: 8.9g Fats: 15.4g Calories: 320

Ingredients:
- Macaroni: 1 cup (after cooking
- Frozen peas: 1 cup rinsed and drained
- Cherry tomatoes: 1 cup diced
- Onions: 1 chopped
- Garlic: 2 cloves
- Vinegar: 3 tbsp
- Olive oil: 2 tbsp
- Tahini: 2 tbsp
- Pepper: as per your taste
- Spring onion greens: 3 tbsp chopped

Directions:
- ❖ Take a pan and heat oil
- ❖ Add onion and sauté for 5 minutes
- ❖ Add tomatoes and whole garlic cloves and sauté for 5 minutes and stir
- ❖ Add in vinegar, tahini, and a lot of pepper
- ❖ Cooking Time: macaroni as per packet instructions and add peas at the end
- ❖ Drain the pasta but keep 2 tablespoons of water and add to tomatoes
- ❖ Add the tomato mixture to the blender and blend
- ❖ Combine pasta and tomato mixture
- ❖ Serve with spring onions on top

36) Brown Rice with Lentils in Veggie Broth

Preparation Time: 5 minutes

Cooking Time: 25 minutes

Servings: 4

Nutrition: Calories: 230 Fat: 8g Carbs: 34g Protein: 8g

Ingredients:
- 2¼ cups low-sodium or no-salt-added vegetable broth
- ½ cup uncooked brown or green lentils
- ½ cup uncooked instant brown rice
- ½ cup diced carrots (about 1 carrot)
- ½ cup diced celery (about 1 stalk)
- 1 (2.25-ounce) can sliced olives, drained (about ½ cup)
- ¼ cup diced red onion (about 1/8 onion)
- ¼ cup chopped fresh curly-leaf parsley
- 1½ tablespoons extra-virgin olive oil
- 1 tablespoon freshly squeezed lemon juice (from about ½ small lemon)
- 1 garlic clove, minced (about ½ teaspoon)
- ¼ teaspoon freshly ground black pepper

Directions:
- ❖ In a medium saucepan over high heat, bring the broth and lentils to a boil, cover, and lower the heat to medium-low. Cook for 8 minutes.
- ❖ Raise the heat to medium, and stir in the rice. Cover the pot and cook the mixture for 15 minutes, or until the liquid is absorbed. Remove the pot from the heat and let it sit, covered, for 1 minute, then stir.
- ❖ While the lentils and rice are cooking, mix together the carrots, celery, olives, onion, and parsley in a large serving bowl.
- ❖ In a small bowl, whisk together the oil, lemon juice, garlic and pepper. Set aside. When the lentils and rice are cooked, add them to the serving bowl.
- ❖ Pour the dressing on top, and mix everything together. Serve warm or cold, or store in a sealed container in the refrigerator for up to 7 days.

37) Golden Rice with Pistachios

Preparation Time: 5 minutes

Cooking Time: 15 minutes

Servings: 6

Nutrition: Calories: 320 **Fat:** 7g **Carbs:** 61g **Protein:** 6g

Ingredients:

- 1 tablespoon extra-virgin olive oil
- 1 cup chopped onion (about ½ medium onion)
- ½ cup shredded carrot (about 1 medium carrot)
- 1 teaspoon ground cumin
- ½ teaspoon ground cinnamon
- 2 cups instant brown rice
- 1¾ cups 100% orange juice
- ¼ cup water
- 1 cup golden raisins
- ½ cup shelled pistachios
- Chopped fresh chives (optional)

Directions:

- ❖ In a medium saucepan over medium-high heat, heat the oil. Add the onion and cook for 5 minutes, stirring frequently.
- ❖ Add the carrot, cumin, and cinnamon, and cook for 1 minute, stirring frequently. Stir in the rice, orange juice, and water.
- ❖ Bring to a boil, cover, then lower the heat to medium-low. Simmer for 7 minutes, or until the rice is cooked through and the liquid is absorbed. Stir in the raisins, pistachios, and chives (if using) and serve.

38) Quinoa and Veggie Mix Salad

Preparation Time: 15 minutes

Cooking Time: 15 minutes

Servings: 4

Nutrition: Calories: 366 Fat: 11.1g Protein: 15.5g Carbs: 55.6g

Ingredients:

- 1 cup red dry quinoa, rinsed and drained
- 2 cups low-sodium vegetable soup
- 2 cups fresh spinach
- 2 cups finely shredded red cabbage
- 1 (15-ounce / 425-g) can chickpeas, drained and rinsed
- 1 ripe avocado, thinly sliced
- 1 cup shredded carrots
- 1 red bell pepper, thinly sliced
- 4 tablespoons Mango Sauce
- ½ cup fresh cilantro, chopped
- Mango Sauce:
- 1 mango, diced
- ¼ cup fresh lime juice
- ½ teaspoon ground turmeric
- 1 teaspoon finely minced fresh ginger
- Pinch of ground red pepper
- 1 teaspoon pure maple syrup
- 2 tablespoons extra-virgin olive oil

Directions:

- ❖ Pour the quinoa and vegetable soup in a saucepan. Bring to a boil. Reduce the heat to low. Cover and cook for 15 minutes or until tender. Fluffy with a fork.
- ❖ Meanwhile, combine the ingredients for the mango sauce in a food processor. Pulse until smooth.
- ❖ Divide the quinoa, spinach, and cabbage into 4 serving bowls, then top with chickpeas, avocado, carrots, and bell pepper.
- ❖ Dress them with the mango sauce and spread with cilantro. Serve immediately.

39) Chili Bean Mix

Preparation Time: 15 minutes

Cooking Time: 5 hours

Servings: 4

Nutrition: Calories: 633 Fat: 16.3g Protein: 31.7g Carbs: 97.0g

Ingredients:

- 1 (28-ounce / 794-g) can chopped tomatoes, with the juice
- 1 (15-ounce / 425-g) can black beans, drained and rinsed
- 1 (15-ounce / 425-g) can redly beans, drained and rinsed
- 1 medium green bell pepper, chopped
- 1 yellow onion, chopped
- 1 tablespoon onion powder
- 1 teaspoon paprika
- 1 teaspoon cayenne pepper
- 1 teaspoon garlic powder
- ½ teaspoon ground black pepper
- 1 tablespoon olive oil
- 1 large hass avocado, pitted, peeled, and chopped, for garnish

Directions:

- ❖ Combine all the ingredients, except for the avocado, in the slow cooker. Stir to mix well.
- ❖ Put the slow cooker lid on and cook on high for 5 hours or until the vegetables are tender and the mixture has a thick consistency.
- ❖ Pour the chili in a large serving bowl. Allow to cool for 30 minutes, then spread with chopped avocado and serve.

40) Bean Balls with Red pepper and Marinara Sauce

Preparation Time: 15 minutes

Cooking Time: 30 minutes

Servings: 2-4

Nutrition: Calories: 351 Fat: 16.4g Protein: 11.5g Carbs: 42.9g

Ingredients:

Bean Balls:
- 1 tablespoon extra-virgin olive oil
- ½ yellow onion, minced
- 1 teaspoon fennel seeds
- 2 teaspoons dried oregano
- ½ teaspoon crushed red pepper flakes
- 1 teaspoon garlic powder
- 1 (15-ounce / 425-g) can white beans (cannellini or navy), drained and rinsed
- ½ cup whole-grain bread crumbs
- Ground black pepper, to taste

Marinara:
- 1 tablespoon extra-virgin olive oil
- 3 garlic cloves, minced
- Handful basil leaves
- 1 (28-ounce / 794-g) can chopped tomatoes with juice reserved

Directions:

- ❖ Preheat the oven to 350°F (180°C). Line a baking sheet with parchment paper. Heat the olive oil in a nonstick skillet over medium heat until shimmering.
- ❖ Add the onion and sauté for 5 minutes or until translucent. Sprinkle with fennel seeds, oregano, red pepper flakes, and garlic powder, then cook for 1 minute or until aromatic.
- ❖ Pour the sautéed mixture in a food processor and add the beans and bread crumbs. Sprinkle with ground black pepper, then pulse to combine well and the mixture holds together.
- ❖ Shape the mixture into balls with a 2-ounce (57-g) cookie scoop, then arrange the balls on the baking sheet.
- ❖ Bake in the preheated oven for 30 minutes or until lightly browned. Flip the balls halfway through the cooking time.
- ❖ While baking the bean balls, heat the olive oil in a saucepan over medium-high heat until shimmering. Add the garlic and basil and sauté for 2 minutes or until fragrant.
- ❖ Fold in the tomatoes and juice. Bring to a boil. Reduce the heat to low. Put the lid on and simmer for 15 minutes.
- ❖ Transfer the bean balls on a large plate and baste with marinara before serving.

Chapter 4 -   Side and Salad Recipes

41) Veggie ChimiSalad

Preparation Time: 10 minutes

Cooking Time: 25 minutes

Servings: 4

Nutrition: Calories 231 Fat 20.1 g Carbs 20.1 g Protein 4.6 g

Ingredients:

- Roasted vegetables:
- 1 large sweet potato (chopped
- 6 red potatoes, quartered
- 2 whole carrots, chopped
- 2 tablespoons melted coconut oil
- 2 teaspoons curry powder
- 1 cup chopped broccolini
- 2 cups red cabbage, chopped
- 1 medium red bell pepper, sliced
- Chimichurri:
- 5 cloves garlic, chopped
- 1 medium serrano pepper
- 1 cup packed cilantro
- 1 cup parsley
- 3 tablespoons ripe avocado
- 3 tablespoons lime juice
- 1 tablespoon maple syrup
- Water to thin
- Salad:
- 4 cups hearty greens
- 1 medium ripe avocado, chopped
- 3 tablespoons hemp seeds
- Fresh herbs
- 5 medium radishes, sliced
- ¼ cup macadamia nut cheese

Directions:

- ❖ Preheat your oven to 400 degrees F.
- ❖ In a suitable bowl, toss all the vegetables for roasting with curry powder and oil.
- ❖ Divide these vegetables into two roasting pans.
- ❖ Bake the vegetables for 25 minutes in the oven.
- ❖ Meanwhile, in a blender, blend all chimichurri sauce ingredients until smooth.
- ❖ In a salad bowl, toss in all the roasted vegetables, chimichurri sauce and salad ingredients.
- ❖ Mix them well then refrigerate to chill.
- ❖ Serve.

42) Exotic Quinoa Bowl

Preparation Time: 15 minutes

Cooking Time: 15 minutes

Servings: 4

Nutrition: Calories: 669 Fat: 40g Protein: 17g Carbs: 69g

Ingredients:

- 1½ cups quinoa
- 2 cucumbers, seeded and diced
- 1 small red onion, diced
- 1 large tomato, diced
- 1 handful fresh flat-leaf parsley, chopped
- ½ cup extra-virgin olive oil
- ¼ cup red wine vinegar
- Juice of 1 lemon
- ¾ teaspoon freshly ground black pepper
- 4 heads endive, trimmed and separated into spears
- 1 avocado, pitted, peeled, and diced

Directions:

- ❖ In a saucepan, prepare the quinoa according to package directions. Rinse the quinoa under cold running water and drain very well. Transfer to a large bowl. Add the cucumbers, red onion, tomato, and parsley.
- ❖ In a small bowl, whisk together the olive oil, vinegar, lemon juice, and pepper. Pour the dressing over the quinoa mixture and toss to coat. Spoon the mixture onto the endive spears and top with the avocado.

43) Linguini with Peas and Parmigiano Reggiano

Preparation Time: 10 minutes

Cooking Time: 10 minutes

Servings: 4

Nutrition: Calories: 480 Protein: 20 g Fat: 11 g Carbs: 73 g

Ingredients:

- 2 eggs
- 1 cup frozen peas
- ½ cup Parmigiano-Reggiano cheese, grated
- 12 ounces linguini
- 1 Tbsp olive oil
- 1 onion, sliced
- Pepper, to taste

Directions:

- ❖ In a bowl, combine the zucchini noodles with pepper and the olive oil and toss well. Prepare linguini according to the package. Whisk eggs and mix in cheese.
- ❖ Sauté onion in olive oil, then stir in peas. Add pasta to pan. Add egg mixture to the pasta and cook for another 2 min. Season with pepper. Serve hot.

44) Noodles Salad with Peanut Butter Cream

Preparation Time: 10 minutes

Cooking Time: 0 minutes

Servings: 04

Nutrition: Calories 361 Fat 16.3 g Carbs 29.3 g Protein 3.3 g

Ingredients:
- Salad:
- 6 ounces vermicelli noodles, boiled
- 2 medium whole carrots, ribboned
- 2 stalks green onions, chopped
- ¼ cup cilantro, chopped
- 2 tablespoons mint, chopped
- 1 cup packed spinach, chopped
- 1 cup red cabbage, sliced
- 1 medium red bell pepper, sliced
- Dressing:
- ⅓ cup creamy peanut butter
- 3 tablespoons tamari
- 3 tablespoons maple syrup
- 1 teaspoon chili garlic sauce
- 1 medium lime, juiced
- ¼ cup water

Directions:
- ❖ Combine all the dressing ingredients in a small bowl.
- ❖ In a salad bowl, toss in the noodles, salad, and dressing.
- ❖ Mix them well then refrigerate to chill.
- ❖ Serve.

45) Delicious Potato Salad with Mustard

Preparation Time: 15 minutes

Cooking Time: 10 minutes

Servings: 4-6

Nutrition: Calories: 140 Carbs: 1g Fat: 15g Protein: 1g

Ingredients:
- ¼ cup extra-virgin olive oil
- ½ teaspoon pepper
- 1 garlic clove, peeled and threaded on skewer
- 1 small shallot, minced
- 1 tablespoon minced fresh chervil
- 1 tablespoon minced fresh chives
- 1 tablespoon minced fresh parsley
- 1 teaspoon minced fresh tarragon
- 1½ tablespoons white wine vinegar or Champagne vinegar
- 2 pounds small red potatoes, unpeeled, sliced ¼ inch thick
- 2 teaspoons Dijon mustard

Directions:
- ❖ Place potatoes in a big saucepan, put in water to cover by 1 inch, and bring to boil on high heat. Put in salt, decrease the heat to simmer, and cook until potatoes are soft and paring knife can be slipped in and out of potatoes with little resistance, about 6 minutes.
- ❖ While potatoes are cooking, lower skewered garlic into simmering water and blanch for 45 seconds. Run garlic under cold running water, then remove from skewer and mince.
- ❖ Reserve ¼ cup cooking water, then drain potatoes and lay out on tight one layer in rimmed baking sheet.
- ❖ Beat oil, minced garlic, vinegar, mustard, pepper, and reserved potato cooking water together in a container, then drizzle over potatoes. Let potatoes sit until flavors blend, about 10 minutes.
- ❖ Move potatoes to big container. Mix shallot and herbs in a small-sized container, then drizzle over potatoes and gently toss to coat using rubber spatula. Serve.

46) Easy Creamy Kernel

Preparation Time: 5minutes

Cooking Time:

Servings: 2

Nutrition: Carbs: 44.5g Protein: 11.5g Fats: 11.4g Calories: 306

Ingredients:
- Frozen peas: 1 cup can washed and drained
- Corn kernel: 2 cups can
- Sesame seeds: 2 tbsp
- Pepper: as per your taste
- Cashew cream: ½ cup

Directions:
- ❖ Combine all the ingredients
- ❖ Serve as the side dish

47) *Green Bean with Walnut Mix*

Preparation Time: 15 minutes

Cooking Time: 15 minutes

Servings: 6-8

Nutrition: Calories: 145 Carbs: 0g Fat: 8g Protein: 0g

Ingredients:

- ¼ cup walnuts
- ½ cup extra-virgin olive oil
- 1 scallion, sliced thin
- 2 garlic cloves, unpeeled
- 2 pounds green beans, trimmed
- 2½ cups fresh cilantro leaves and stems, tough stem ends trimmed (about 2 bunches)
- 4 teaspoons lemon juice

Directions:

- ❖ Cook walnuts and garlic in 8-inch frying pan on moderate heat, stirring frequently, until toasted and aromatic, 5 to 7 minutes; move to a container. Let garlic cool slightly, then peel and approximately chop.
- ❖ Process walnuts, garlic, cilantro, oil, lemon juice, scallion, and 1/8 teaspoon pepper using a food processor until smooth, about 1 minute, scraping down sides of the container as required; move to big container.
- ❖ Bring 4 quarts water to boil in large pot on high heat. In the meantime, fill big container halfway with ice and water.
- ❖ Put in green beans to boiling water and cook until crisp-tender, 3 to 5 minutes. Drain green beans, move to ice water, and allow to sit until chilled, approximately two minutes.
- ❖ Move green beans to a container with cilantro sauce and gently toss until coated. Sprinkle with pepper to taste. Serve.

48) *Old School Panzanella*

Preparation Time: 15 minutes

Cooking Time: 20 minutes

Servings: 6

Nutrition: Calories: 294 Carbs: 32g Fat: 15g Protein: 9g

Ingredients:

- 1 (15-ounce) can cannellini beans, rinsed
- 1 small red onion, halved and sliced thin
- 1½ pounds ripe tomatoes, cored and chopped, seeds and juice reserved
- 12 ounces rustic Italian bread, cut into 1-inch pieces (4 cups)
- 2 ounces Parmesan cheese, shaved
- 2 tablespoons minced fresh oregano
- 3 ounces (3 cups) baby arugula
- 3 tablespoons chopped fresh basil
- 3 tablespoons red wine vinegar
- 5 tablespoons extra-virgin olive oil

Directions:

- ❖ Place the oven rack in the center of the oven and pre-heat your oven to 350 degrees. Toss bread pieces with 1 tablespoon oil and sprinkle with pepper.
- ❖ Arrange bread in one layer in rimmed baking sheet and bake, stirring intermittently, until light golden brown, fifteen to twenty minutes. Allow it to cool to room temperature.
- ❖ Beat vinegar in a big container. Whisking continuously, slowly drizzle in remaining ¼ cup oil.
- ❖ Put in tomatoes with their seeds and juice, beans, onion, 1½ tablespoons basil, and 1 tablespoon oregano, toss to coat, and allow to sit for 20 minutes.
- ❖ Put in cooled croutons, arugula, remaining 1½ tablespoons basil, and remaining 1 tablespoon oregano and gently toss to combine.
- ❖ Sprinkle with pepper to taste. Move salad to serving platter and drizzle with Parmesan. Serve.

49) *Vegan Chorizo Salad with Red Wine Vinegar*

Preparation Time: 5 minutes

Cooking Time: 5 minutes

Servings: 4

Nutrition: Calories 138, Fat 8.95g, Carbs 5.63g, Protein 7.12g

Ingredients:

- 2 ½ tbsp olive oil
- 4 soy chorizo, chopped
- 2 tsp red wine vinegar
- 1 small red onion, finely chopped
- 2 ½ cups cherry tomatoes, halved
- 2 tbsp chopped cilantro
- Freshly ground black pepper to taste
- 3 tbsp sliced black olives to garnish

Directions:

- ❖ Over medium fire, heat half tablespoon of olive oil in a skillet and fry soy chorizo until golden. Turn heat off.
- ❖ In a salad bowl, whisk remaining olive oil and vinegar. Add onion, cilantro, tomatoes, and soy chorizo. Mix with dressing and season with black pepper.
- ❖ Garnish with olives and serve.

50) *Juicy Smoked Apple Salad*

Preparation Time: 15 minutes

Cooking Time: 0 minutes

Servings: 4-6

Nutrition: Calories: 157 Carbs: 12g Fat: 13g Protein: 1g

Ingredients:

- ¼ cup extra-virgin olive oil
- 1 fennel bulb, stalks discarded, bulb halved, cored, and sliced thin
- 1 small shallot, minced
- 1 tablespoon whole-grain mustard
- 2 Granny Smith apples, peeled, cored, and cut into 3-inch-long matchsticks
- 2 teaspoons minced fresh tarragon
- 3 tablespoons lemon juice
- 5 ounces (5 cups) watercress
- 6 ounces smoked mackerel, skin and pin bones removed, flaked
- Pepper

Directions:

- ❖ Beat lemon juice, mustard, shallot, 1 teaspoon tarragon, and ¼ teaspoon pepper together in a big container.
- ❖ Whisking continuously, slowly drizzle in oil. Put in watercress, apples, and fennel and gently toss to coat. Sprinkle with pepper to taste.
- ❖ Divide salad among plates and top with flaked mackerel. Sprinkle any remaining dressing over mackerel and drizzle with remaining 1 teaspoon tarragon. Serve instantly.

51) *Kalamata Pepper Salad with Pine Nuts*

Preparation Time: 10 minutes

Cooking Time: 20 minutes

Servings: 4

Nutrition: Calories 163, Fat 13.3g, Carbs 6.53g, Protein 3.37g

Ingredients:

- 8 large red bell peppers, deseeded and cut in wedges
- ½ tsp erythritol
- 2 ½ tbsp olive oil
- 1/3 cup arugula
- 1 tbsp mint leaves
- 1/3 cup pitted Kalamata olives
- 3 tbsp chopped almonds
- ½ tbsp balsamic vinegar
- Crumbled feta cheese for topping
- Toasted pine nuts for topping

Directions:

- ❖ Preheat oven to 400o F.
- ❖ Pour bell peppers on a roasting pan; season with erythritol and drizzle with half of olive oil. Roast in oven until slightly charred, 20 minutes. Remove from oven and set aside.
- ❖ Arrange arugula in a salad bowl, scatter bell peppers on top, mint leaves, olives, almonds, and drizzle with balsamic vinegar and remaining olive oil. Season with black pepper.
- ❖ Toss; top with feta cheese and pine nuts and serve.

52) *Spiced Carrot Bowl*

Preparation Time: 15 minutes

Cooking Time: 0 minutes

Servings: 4-6

Nutrition: Calories: 84 Carbs: 13g Fat: 4g Protein: 1g

Ingredients:

- 1/8 teaspoon cayenne pepper
- 1/8 teaspoon ground cinnamon
- ¾ teaspoon ground cumin
- 1-pound carrots, peeled and shredded
- 1 tablespoon lemon juice
- 1 teaspoon honey
- 2 oranges
- 3 tablespoons extra-virgin olive oil
- 3 tablespoons minced fresh cilantro

Directions:

- ❖ Cut away peel and pith from oranges. Holding fruit over bowl, use paring knife to slice between membranes to release segments.
- ❖ Cut segments in half crosswise and allow to drain in fine-mesh strainer set over big container, reserving juice.
- ❖ Beat lemon juice, honey, cumin, cayenne, cinnamon into reserved orange juice.
- ❖ Put in drained oranges and carrots and gently toss to coat. Allow to sit until liquid starts to pool in bottom of bowl, 3 to 5 minutes.
- ❖ Drain salad in fine-mesh strainer and return to now-empty bowl. Mix in cilantro and oil and sprinkle with pepper to taste. Serve.

53) *Double Green Juicy Salad*

Preparation Time: 10 minutes

Cooking Time: 15 minutes

Servings: 4

Nutrition: Calories 237, Fat 19.57g, Carbs 5.9g, Protein 12.75g

Ingredients:

- 1 (7 ozblock extra firm tofu
- 2 tbsp olive oil
- 2 tbsp butter
- 1 cup asparagus, trimmed and halved
- 1 cup green beans, trimmed
- 2 tbsp chopped dulse
- Freshly ground black pepper to taste
- ½ lemon, juiced
- 4 tbsp chopped walnuts

Directions:

- ❖ Place tofu in between two paper towels and allow soaking for 5 minutes. After, remove towels and chop into small cubes.
- ❖ Heat olive oil in a skillet and fry tofu until golden, 10 minutes. Remove onto a paper towel-lined plate and set aside.
- ❖ Melt butter in skillet and sauté asparagus
- ❖ And green beans until softened, 5 minutes. Add dulse, season with black pepper, and Cooking Time: until softened. Mix in tofu and stir-fry for 5 minutes.
- ❖ Plate, drizzle with lemon juice, and scatter walnuts on top.
- ❖ Serve warm.

54) *Lemony Orange Fennel Salad*

Preparation Time: 15 minutes

Cooking Time: 0 minutes

Servings: 4-6

Nutrition: Calories: 180 Carbs: 21g Fat: 11g Protein: 3g

Ingredients:

- ¼ cup coarsely chopped fresh mint
- ¼ cup extra-virgin olive oil
- ½ cup pitted oil-cured black olives, quartered
- 2 fennel bulbs, stalks discarded, bulbs halved, cored, and sliced thin
- 2 tablespoons lemon juice
- 4 blood oranges
- Pepper

Directions:

❖ Cut away peel and pith from oranges. Quarter oranges, then slice crosswise into ¼-inch-thick pieces. Mix oranges, fennel, olives, and mint in a big container.

❖ Beat lemon juice, and 1/8 teaspoon pepper together in a small-sized container. Whisking continuously, slowly drizzle in oil.

❖ Sprinkle dressing over salad and gently toss to coat. Sprinkle with pepper to taste. Serve.

55) *Asian Goji Salad*

Preparation Time: 10 minutes

Cooking Time: 2 minutes

Servings: 4

Nutrition: Calories 203, Fat 15.28g, Carbs 9.64g, Protein 6.67g, Protein 2.54g

Ingredients:

- 1 small head cauliflower, cut into florets
- 8 sun-dried tomatoes in olive oil, drained
- 12 pitted green olives, roughly chopped
- 1 lemon, zested and juiced
- 3 tbsp chopped green onions
- A handful chopped almonds
- ¼ cup goji berries
- 1 tbsp sesame oil
- ½ cup watercress
- 3 tbsp chopped parsley
- Freshly ground black pepper to taste
- Lemon wedges to garnish

Directions:

❖ Pour cauliflower into a large safe-microwave bowl, sprinkle with some water, and steam in microwave for 1 to 2 minutes or until softened.

❖ In a large salad bowl, combine cauliflower, tomatoes, olives, lemon zest and juice, green onions, almonds, goji berries, sesame oil, watercress, and parsley. Season with black pepper, and mix well.

❖ Serve with lemon wedges.

56) *Cheesy Asparagus Pesto Salad*

Preparation Time: 15 minutes

Cooking Time: 0 minutes

Servings: 4-6

Nutrition: Calories: 220 Carbs: 40g Fat: 5g Protein: 6g

Ingredients:

Pesto:
- ¼ cup fresh basil leaves
- ¼ cup grated Pecorino Romano cheese
- ½ cup extra-virgin olive oil
- 1 garlic clove, minced
- 1 teaspoon grated lemon zest plus 2 teaspoons juice
- 2 cups fresh mint leaves
- Pepper

Salad:
- ¾ cup hazelnuts, toasted, skinned, and chopped
- 2 oranges
- 2 pounds asparagus, trimmed
- 4 ounces feta cheese, crumbled (1 cup)
- Pepper

Directions:

❖ For the Pesto, process mint, basil, Pecorino, lemon zest and juice, garlic, and ¾ teaspoon salt using a food processor until finely chopped, approximately half a minute, scraping down sides of the container as required. Move to big container. Mix in oil and sprinkle with pepper to taste.

❖ For the Salad, chop asparagus tips from stalks into ¾-inch-long pieces. Cut asparagus stalks 1/8 inch thick on bias into approximate 2-inch lengths.

❖ Cut away the peel and pith from oranges. Holding fruit over bowl, use paring knife to cut between membranes to release segments.

❖ Put in asparagus tips and stalks, orange segments, feta, and hazelnuts to pesto and toss to combine. Sprinkle with pepper to taste. Serve.

57) *Ricotta Seed Salad*

Preparation Time: 15 minutes

Cooking Time:

Servings: 4

Nutrition: Calories 397, Fat 3.87g, Carbs 8.4g, Protein 8.93g

Ingredients:

- 2 tbsp olive oil
- 1 tbsp white wine vinegar
- 2 tbsp chia seeds
- Freshly ground black pepper to taste
- 2 cups broccoli slaw
- 1 cup chopped kelp, thoroughly washed and steamed
- 1/3 cup chopped pecans
- 1/3 cup pumpkin seeds
- 1/3 cup blueberries
- 2/3 cup ricotta cheese

Directions:

❖ In a small bowl, whisk olive oil, white wine vinegar, chia seeds, and black pepper. Set aside.

❖ In a large salad bowl, combine the broccoli slaw, kelp, pecans, pumpkin seeds, blueberries, and ricotta cheese.

❖ Drizzle dressing on top, toss, and serve.

58) Veggie Almond Chermoula Bowl

Preparation Time: 15 minutes

Cooking Time: 22 minutes

Servings: 4-6

Nutrition: Calories: 450 Carbs: 77g Fat: 7g Protein: 20g

Ingredients:

Salad:
- ½ cup raisins
- ½ red onion, sliced ¼ inch thick
- 1 cup shredded carrot
- 1 head cauliflower (2 pounds), cored and cut into 2-inch florets
- 2 tablespoons chopped fresh cilantro
- 2 tablespoons extra-virgin olive oil
- 2 tablespoons sliced almonds, toasted
- Pepper

Chermoula:
- 1/8 teaspoon cayenne pepper
- ¼ cup extra-virgin olive oil
- ½ teaspoon ground cumin
- ½ teaspoon paprika
- ¾ cup fresh cilantro leaves
- 2 tablespoons lemon juice
- 4 garlic cloves, minced

Directions:

- ❖ For the salad, place oven rack to lowest position and pre-heat your oven to 475 degrees. Toss cauliflower with oil and sprinkle with pepper.
- ❖ Arrange cauliflower in one layer in parchment paper–lined rimmed baking sheet. Cover tightly with aluminum foil and roast till they become tender, 5 to 7 minutes.
- ❖ Remove foil and spread onion evenly in sheet. Roast until vegetables are tender, cauliflower becomes deeply golden brown, and onion slices are charred at edges, 10 to 15 minutes, stirring halfway through roasting. Allow it to cool slightly, approximately five minutes.
- ❖ For the chermoula, process all ingredients using a food processor until smooth, about 1 minute, scraping down sides of the container as required. Move to big container.
- ❖ Gently toss cauliflower-onion mixture, carrot, raisins, and cilantro with chermoula until coated. Move to serving platter and drizzle with almonds. Serve warm or at room temperature.

59) Baked Asparagus Maple Salad

Preparation Time: 10 minutes

Cooking Time: 20 minutes

Servings: 4

Nutrition: Calories 146, Fat 12.87g, Carbs 5.07g, Protein 4.44g

Ingredients:

- 1 lb asparagus, trimmed and halved
- 2 tbsp olive oil
- ½ tsp dried basil
- ½ tsp dried oregano
- Freshly ground black pepper to taste
- ½ tsp hemp seeds
- 1 tbsp maple (sugar-freesyrup
- ½ cup arugula
- 4 tbsp crumbled feta cheese
- 2 tbsp hazelnuts
- 1 lemon, cut into wedges

Directions:

- ❖ Preheat oven to 350oF.
- ❖ Pour asparagus on a baking tray, drizzle with olive oil, basil, oregano, black pepper, and hemp seeds. Mix with your hands and roast in oven for 15 minutes.
- ❖ Remove, drizzle with maple syrup, and continue cooking until slightly charred, 5 minutes.
- ❖ Spread arugula in a salad bowl and top with asparagus. Scatter with feta cheese, hazelnuts, and serve with lemon wedges.

60) Cherry Kalamata Salad with Oregano

Preparation Time: 15 minutes

Cooking Time: 10 minutes

Servings: 4-6

Nutrition: Calories: 110 Carbs: 20g Fat: 4g Protein: 1g

Ingredients:

- ½ cup pitted kalamata olives, chopped
- ½ teaspoon sugar
- 1 shallot, minced
- 1 small cucumber, peeled, halved along the length, seeded, and cut into ½-inch pieces
- 1 tablespoon red wine vinegar
- 1½ pounds cherry tomatoes, quartered
- 2 garlic cloves, minced
- 2 tablespoons extra-virgin olive oil
- 2 teaspoons minced fresh oregano
- 3 tablespoons chopped fresh parsley
- 4 ounces feta cheese, crumbled (1 cup)
- Pepper

Directions:

- ❖ Toss tomatoes with sugar and ¼ teaspoon salt in a container and allow to sit for 30 minutes.
- ❖ Move tomatoes to salad spinner and spin until seeds and excess liquid have been removed, 45 to 60 seconds, stopping to redistribute tomatoes several times during spinning.
- ❖ Put in tomatoes, cucumber, olives, feta, and parsley to big container; set aside.
- ❖ Strain ½ cup tomato liquid through fine-mesh strainer into liquid measuring cup; discard remaining liquid.
- ❖ Bring tomato liquid, shallot, vinegar, garlic, and oregano to simmer in small saucepan on moderate heat and cook until reduced to 3 tablespoons, 6 to 8 minutes.
- ❖ Move to small-sized container and allow to cool to room temperature, approximately five minutes. Whisking continuously, slowly drizzle in oil.
- ❖ Sprinkle dressing over salad and gently toss to coat. Sprinkle with pepper to taste. Serve.

Chapter 5 -   Main Recipes

61) Zucchini Rice with Chicken Chunks

Preparation Time: 10 minutes

Cooking Time: 14 minutes

Servings: 4

Nutrition: Calories 500 Fat 16.5 g Carbs 48 g Protein 38.7 g

Ingredients:

- 3 chicken breasts, skinless, boneless, and cut into chunks
- 1/4 fresh parsley, chopped
- 1 zucchini, sliced
- 2 bell peppers, chopped
- 1 cup rice, rinsed and drained
- 1 1/2 cup chicken broth
- 1 tbsp oregano
- 3 tbsp fresh lemon juice
- 1 tbsp garlic, minced
- 1 onion, diced
- 2 tbsp olive oil
- Pepper

Directions:

- Add oil into the inner pot of instant pot and set the pot on sauté mode. Add onion and chicken and cook for 5 minutes. Add rice, oregano, lemon juice, garlic, broth, pepper, and stir everything well.
- Seal pot with lid and cook on high for 4 minutes. Once done, release pressure using quick release. Remove lid. Add parsley, zucchini, and bell peppers and stir well.
- Seal pot again with lid and select manual and set timer for 5 minutes. Release pressure using quick release. Remove lid. Stir well and serve.

62) Smoked Baby Spinach Stew

Preparation Time: 10 minutes

Cooking Time: 25 minutes

Servings: 4

Nutrition: Calories 369 Fat 9.7g Carbs 67.9g Protein 18g

Ingredients:

- 1 splash olive oil
- 1 small onion, chopped
- 2 cloves garlic
- 5g cumin powder
- 5g smoked paprika
- ¼ teaspoon chili powder
- 235ml water
- 670g can diced tomatoes
- 165g cooked chickpeas (or can chickpeas
- 60g baby spinach
- A handful of chopped coriander, to garnish
- 20g slivered almonds, to garnish
- 4 slices toasted whole-grain bread, to serve

Directions:

- Heat olive oil in a saucepan over medium-high heat.
- Add onion and Cooking Time: until browned, for 7-8 minutes.
- Add garlic, cumin, paprika, and chili powder.
- Cooking Time: 1 minute.
- Add water and scrape any browned bits.
- Add the tomatoes and chickpeas. Season to taste and reduce heat.
- Simmer the soup for 10 minutes.
- Stir in spinach and Cooking Time: 2 minutes.
- Ladle soup in a bowl. Sprinkle with cilantro and almonds.
- Serve with toasted bread slices.

63) Green Chilis Chicken Breast

Preparation Time: 10 minutes

Cooking Time: 10 minutes

Servings: 3

Nutrition: Calories 237 Fat 8 g Carbs 10.8 g Protein 30.5 g

Ingredients:

- 2 chicken breasts, skinless and boneless
- 1 tbsp chili powder
- 1/2 tsp ground cumin
- 1/2 tsp garlic powder
- 1/4 tsp onion powder
- 1/2 tsp paprika
- 4 oz can green chilis, diced
- 1/4 cup chicken broth
- 14 oz can tomato, diced
- Pepper

Directions:

- Add all ingredients except chicken into the instant pot and stir well. Add chicken and stir. Seal pot with lid and cook on high for 10 minutes.
- Once done, allow to release pressure naturally for 5 minutes then release remaining using quick release. Remove lid.
- Remove chicken from pot and shred using a fork. Return shredded chicken to the pot and stir well. Serve and enjoy.

64) Chicken Breast with Italian Seasoning

Preparation Time: 10 minutes

Cooking Time: 12 minutes

Servings: 8

Nutrition: Calories 502 Fat 20 g Carbs 7.8 g Protein 66.8 g

Ingredients:

- 4 lb. chicken breasts, skinless and boneless
- 1 tbsp garlic powder
- 2 tbsp dried Italian herb mix
- 2 tbsp olive oil
- 1/4 cup chicken stock
- Pepper

Directions:

- Coat chicken with oil and season with dried herb, garlic powder, pepper. Place chicken into the instant pot. Pour stock over the chicken. Seal pot with a lid and select manual and set timer for 12 minutes.
- Once done, allow to release pressure naturally for 5 minutes then release remaining using quick release. Remove lid. Shred chicken using a fork and serve.

65) Veggie Ragù Noodles

Preparation Time: 10 minutes

Cooking Time: 15 minutes (plus 25 for lentils

Servings: 4

Nutrition: Calories 353 Fat 0.9g Carbs 74g Protein 17.7g

Ingredients:
- Bolognese:
- 100g red lentils
- 1 bay leaf
- Splash of olive oil
- 1 small onion, diced
- 1 large stalk celery, sliced
- 3 cloves garlic, minced
- 230ml tomato sauce or fresh pureed tomatoes
- 60ml red wine or vegetable stock (if you do not like wine)
- 1 tablespoon fresh basil, chopped
- Pepper, to taste
- Soba noodles:
- 280g soba noodles

Directions:
- ❖ Cooking Time: the lentils; place lentils and bay leaf in a saucepan.
- ❖ Cover with water, so the water is 2-inches above the lentils.
- ❖ Bring to a boil over medium-high heat.
- ❖ Reduce heat and simmer the lentils for 25 minutes.
- ❖ Drain the lentils and discard the bay leaf.
- ❖ Heat a splash of olive oil in a saucepan.
- ❖ Add onion, and Cooking Time: 6 minutes.
- ❖ Add celery and Cooking Time: 2 minutes.
- ❖ Add garlic and Cooking Time: 2 minutes.
- ❖ Add the tomatoes and wine. Simmer the mixture for 5 minutes.
- ❖ Stir in the lentils and simmer 2 minutes.
- ❖ Remove the Bolognese from the heat and stir in basil.
- ❖ In the meantime, Cooking Time: the soba noodles according to package directions.
- ❖ Serve noodles with lentils Bolognese.

66) Quinoa Chicken with Olives and Grrek Seasoning

Preparation Time: 10 minutes

Cooking Time: 6 minutes

Servings: 4

Nutrition: Calories 566 Fat 16.4 g Carbs 57.4 g Protein 46.8 g

Ingredients:
- 1 lb. chicken breasts, skinless, boneless, and cut into chunks
- 14 oz can chickpeas, drained and rinsed
- 1 cup olives, pitted and sliced
- 1 cup cherry tomatoes, halved
- 1 cucumber, sliced
- 2 tsp Greek seasoning
- 1 1/2 cups chicken broth
- 1 cup quinoa, rinsed and drained
- Pepper

Directions:
- ❖ Add broth and quinoa into the instant pot and stir well. Season chicken with Greek seasoning, pepper and place into the instant pot.
- ❖ Seal pot with lid and cook on high for 6 minutes. Once done, release pressure using quick release. Remove lid. Stir quinoa and chicken mixture well.
- ❖ Add remaining ingredients and stir everything well. Serve immediately and enjoy it.

67) Red Quinoa Burgers with Thaini Guacamole

Preparation Time: 10 minutes

Cooking Time: 50 minutes

Servings: 4

Nutrition: Calories 343 Fat 16.6g Total Carbs 49.1g Protein 15g

Ingredients:
- Patties:
- 2 large beets, peeled, cubed
- 1 red onion, cut into chunks
- 115g red kidney beans
- 85g red cooked quinoa
- 2 cloves garlic, minced
- 30g almond meal
- 20g ground flax
- 10ml lemon juice
- ½ teaspoon ground cumin
- ½ teaspoon red pepper flakes
- 4 whole-meal burger buns
- Tahini Guacamole:
- 1 avocado, pitted, peeled
- 45ml lime juice
- 30g tahini sauce
- 5g chopped coriander

Directions:
- ❖ Preheat oven to 190C/375F.
- ❖ Toss beet and onion with a splash of olive oil.
- ❖ Bake the beets for 30 minutes.
- ❖ Transfer the beets and onion into a food blender.
- ❖ Add the beans and blend until coarse. You do not want a completely smooth mixture.
- ❖ Stir in quinoa, garlic, almond meal, flax seeds, lemon juice, cumin, and red pepper flakes.
- ❖ Shape the mixture into four patties.
- ❖ Transfer the patties to a baking sheet, lined with parchment paper.
- ❖ Bake the patties 20 minutes, flipping halfway through.
- ❖ In the meantime, make the tahini guac; mash the avocado with lime juice in a bowl.
- ❖ Stir in tahini and coriander. Season to taste.
- ❖ To serve; place the patty in the bun, top with guacamole and serve.

68) Rice and Beans with Red Bell pepper

Preparation Time: 10 minutes

Cooking Time: 1 hour 10 minutes

Servings: 6

Nutrition: Calories 469 Fat 6g Carbs 87.5g Protein 21.1g

Ingredients:
- 450g dry red kidney beans, soaked overnight
- 15ml olive oil
- 1 onion, diced
- 1 red bell pepper, seeded, diced
- 1 large stalk celery, sliced
- 4 cloves garlic, minced
- 15ml hot sauce
- 5g paprika
- 2g dried thyme
- 2 g parsley, chopped
- 2 bay leaves
- 900ml vegetable stock
- 280g brown rice
- Pepper, to taste

Directions:
- ❖ Drain the beans and place aside.
- ❖ Heat olive oil in a saucepot.
- ❖ Add onion and bell pepper. Cooking Time: 6 minutes.
- ❖ Add celery and Cooking Time: 3 minutes.
- ❖ Add garlic, hot sauce, paprika, and thyme. Cooking Time: 1 minute.
- ❖ Add the drained beans, bay leaves, and vegetable stock.
- ❖ Bring to a boil, and reduce heat.
- ❖ Simmer the beans for 1 hour 15 minutes or until tender.
- ❖ In the meantime, place rice in a small saucepot. Cover the rice with 4cm water.
- ❖ Season to taste and Cooking Time: the rice until tender, for 25 minutes.
- ❖ To serve; transfer ¼ of the beans into a food processor. Process until smooth.
- ❖ Combine the processed beans with the remaining beans and ladle into a bowl.
- ❖ Add rice and sprinkle with parsley before serving.

69) Baked Sole with Pistachos

Preparation Time: 5 minutes

Cooking Time: 10 minutes

Servings: 2

Nutrition: 166 Calories 6g Fat 2g Carbs 6g Protein

Ingredients:
- 4 (5 ounces) boneless sole fillets
- ½ cup pistachios, finely chopped
- Juice of 1 lemon
- teaspoon extra virgin olive oil

Directions:
- ❖ Pre-heat your oven to 350 degrees Fahrenheit
- ❖ Wrap baking sheet using parchment paper and keep it on the side
- ❖ Pat fish dry with kitchen towels and lightly season with salt and pepper
- ❖ Take a small bowl and stir in pistachios
- ❖ Place sol on the prepped sheet and press 2 tablespoons of pistachio mixture on top of each fillet
- ❖ Rub the fish with lemon juice and olive oil
- ❖ Bake for 10 minutes until the top is golden and fish flakes with a fork

70) Quinoa with Avocado and Pepper Mix

Preparation Time: 15 minutes

Cooking Time: 1 hour 5 minutes

Servings: 4

Nutrition: Calories 456 Total Fat 15.4g Carbs 71.1g Protein 8g

Ingredients:
- 160g quinoa
- 460ml vegetable stock
- 2 red bell peppers, cut in half, seeds and membrane removed
- 2 yellow bell peppers, cut in half, seeds, and membrane removed
- 120g salsa
- 15g nutritional yeast
- 10g chili powder
- 5g cumin powder
- 425g can black beans, rinsed, drained
- 160g fresh corn kernels
- Pepper, to taste
- 1 small avocado, sliced
- 15g chopped cilantro

Directions:
- ❖ Preheat oven to 190C/375F.
- ❖ Brush the baking sheet with some cooking oil.
- ❖ Combine quinoa and vegetable stock in a saucepan. Bring to a boil.
- ❖ Reduce heat and simmer 20 minutes.
- ❖ Transfer the quinoa to a large bowl.
- ❖ Stir in salsa, nutritional yeast, chili powder, cumin powder, black beans, and corn. Season to taste with pepper.
- ❖ Stuff the bell pepper halves with prepared mixture.
- ❖ Transfer the peppers onto a baking sheet, cover with aluminum foil, and bake for 30 minutes.
- ❖ Increase heat to 200C/400F and bake the peppers for an additional 15 minutes.
- ❖ Serve warm, topped with avocado slices, and chopped cilantro.

71) Lemony Mussels in Dry Wine Sauce

Preparation Time: 5 minutes

Cooking Time: 10 minutes

Servings: 2

Nutrition: Calories 22, 7 g fat, 1 g fiber, 18 g protein

Ingredients:

- 2 pounds small mussels
- 1 tablespoon extra-virgin olive oil
- 1 cup thinly sliced red onion
- 3 garlic cloves, sliced
- 1 cup dry white wine
- 2 (¼-inch-thick) lemon slices
- ¼ teaspoon freshly ground black pepper
- Fresh lemon wedges, for serving (optional)

Directions:

- ❖ In a large colander in the sink, run cold water over the mussels (but don't let the mussels sit in standing water).
- ❖ All the shells should be closed tight; discard any shells that are a little bit open or any shells that are cracked. Leave the mussels in the colander until you're ready to use them.
- ❖ In a large skillet over medium-high heat, heat the oil. Add the onion and cook for 4 minutes, stirring occasionally.
- ❖ Add the garlic and cook for 1 minute, stirring constantly. Add the wine, lemon slices, pepper, and bring to a simmer. Cook for 2 minutes.
- ❖ Add the mussels and cover. Cook for 3 minutes, or until the mussels open their shells. Gently shake the pan two or three times while they are cooking.
- ❖ All the shells should now be wide open. Using a slotted spoon, discard any mussels that are still closed. Spoon the opened mussels into a shallow serving bowl, and pour the broth over the top. Serve with additional fresh lemon slices, if desired.

72) Cold Spinach with Fruit Mix

Preparation Time: 5 minutes

Cooking Time: 0 minute

Servings: 1

Nutrition: Calories 296 Fat 18 g Carbs 27 g Protein 8 g

Ingredients:

- 3 cups baby spinach
- ½ cup strawberries, sliced
- 1 tablespoon white onion, chopped
- 2 tablespoons vinaigrette
- ¼ medium avocado, diced
- 2 tablespoons walnut, toasted

Directions:

- ❖ Put the spinach, strawberries and onion in a glass jar with lid.
- ❖ Drizzle dressing on top.
- ❖ Top with avocado and walnuts.
- ❖ Seal the lid and refrigerate until ready to serve.

73) Juiced Shrimp with Herbs

Preparation Time: 20 minutes

Cooking Time: 10 minutes

Servings: 2

Nutrition: Calories 190, 8 g fat, 1 g fiber, 24 g protein

Ingredients:

- 1 large orange
- 3 tablespoons extra-virgin olive oil, divided
- 1 tablespoon chopped fresh Rosemary
- 1 tablespoon chopped fresh thyme
- 3 garlic cloves, minced (about 1½ teaspoons)
- ¼ teaspoon freshly ground black pepper
- 1½ pounds fresh raw shrimp, shells, and tails removed

Directions:

- ❖ Zest the entire orange using a citrus grater. In a large zip-top plastic bag, combine the orange zest and 2 tablespoons of oil with the Rosemary, thyme, garlic and pepper
- ❖ Add the shrimp, seal the bag, and gently massage the shrimp until all the ingredients are combined and the shrimp is completely covered with the seasonings. Set aside.
- ❖ Heat a grill, grill pan, or a large skillet over medium heat. Brush on or swirl in the remaining 1 tablespoon of oil.
- ❖ Add half the shrimp, and cook for 4 to 6 minutes, or until the shrimp turn pink and white, flipping halfway through if on the grill or stirring every minute if in a pan. Transfer the shrimp to a large serving bowl.
- ❖ Repeat with the remaining shrimp, and add them to the bowl.
- ❖ While the shrimp cook, peel the orange and cut the flesh into bite-size pieces. Add to the serving bowl, and toss with the cooked shrimp. Serve immediately or refrigerate and serve cold.

74) Veggie Grill with Herbs and Cider Vinegar

Preparation Time: 15 minutes

Cooking Time: 6 minutes

Servings: 6

Nutrition: Calories 127 Fat 9 g Carbs 11 g Protein 3 g

Ingredients:

- 2 teaspoons cider vinegar
- 1 tablespoon olive oil
- ¼ teaspoon fresh thyme, chopped
- 1 teaspoon fresh parsley, chopped
- ¼ teaspoon fresh rosemary, chopped
- Pepper to taste
- 1 onion, sliced into wedges
- 2 red bell peppers, sliced
- 3 tomatoes, sliced in half
- 6 large mushrooms, stems removed
- 1 eggplant, sliced crosswise
- 3 tablespoons olive oil
- 1 tablespoon cider vinegar

Directions:

- ❖ Make the dressing by mixing the vinegar, oil, thyme, parsley, rosemary and pepper.
- ❖ In a bowl, mix the onion, red bell pepper, tomatoes, mushrooms and eggplant.
- ❖ Toss in remaining olive oil and cider vinegar.
- ❖ Grill over medium heat for 3 minutes.
- ❖ Turn the vegetables and grill for another 3 minutes.
- ❖ Arrange grilled vegetables in a food container.
- ❖ Drizzle with the herbed mixture when ready to serve.

75) Cheesy Gnocchi with Shrimp

Preparation Time: 10 minutes

Cooking Time: 20 minutes

Servings: 2

Nutrition: Calories 227, 7 g total fat, 1 g fiber, 20 g protein

Ingredients:

- 1 cup chopped fresh tomato
- 2 tablespoons extra-virgin olive oil
- 2 garlic cloves, minced
- ½ teaspoon freshly ground black pepper
- ¼ teaspoon crushed red pepper
- 1 (12-ounces) jar roasted red peppers
- 1-pound fresh raw shrimp, shells and tails removed
- 1-pound frozen gnocchi (not thawed)
- ½ cup cubed feta cheese
- 1/3 cup fresh torn basil leaves

Directions:

- ❖ Preheat the oven to 425°F. In a baking dish, mix the tomatoes, oil, garlic, black pepper, and crushed red pepper. Roast in the oven for 10 minutes.
- ❖ Stir in the roasted peppers and shrimp. Roast for 10 more minutes, until the shrimp turn pink and white.
- ❖ While the shrimp cooks, cook the gnocchi on the stovetop according to the package directions.
- ❖ Drain in a colander and keep warm. Remove the dish from the oven. Mix in the cooked gnocchi, feta, and basil, and serve.

76) Hummus Quinoa with Edamame Bowl

Preparation Time: 10 minutes

Cooking Time: 10 minutes

Servings: 4

Nutrition: Calories 381 Fat 19 g Carbs 43 g Protein 16 g

Ingredients:

- 8 oz. microwavable quinoa
- 2 tablespoons lemon juice
- ½ cup hummus
- Water
- 5 oz. baby kale
- 8 oz. cooked baby beets, sliced
- 1 cup frozen shelled edamame (thawed
- ¼ cup sunflower seeds, toasted
- 1 avocado, sliced
- 1 cup pecans
- 2 tablespoons flaxseeds

Directions:

- ❖ Cooking Time: quinoa according to directions in the packaging.
- ❖ Set aside and let cool.
- ❖ In a bowl, mix the lemon juice and hummus.
- ❖ Add water to achieve desired consistency.
- ❖ Divide mixture into 4 condiment containers.
- ❖ Cover containers with lids and put in the refrigerator.
- ❖ Divide the baby kale into 4 food containers with lids.
- ❖ Top with quinoa, beets, edamame and sunflower seeds.
- ❖ Store in the refrigerator until ready to serve.
- ❖ Before serving add avocado slices and hummus dressing.

77) Fresh Salmon Fillet with Pepper

Preparation Time: 5 minutes

Cooking Time: 2 hours

Servings: 2

Nutrition: Calories 446, 20g fat, 65g protein

Ingredients:

- 2 (6-ounce / 170-g) salmon fillets
- 1 tablespoon olive oil
- 2 cloves garlic, minced
- ½ tablespoon lime juice
- 1 teaspoon finely chopped fresh parsley
- ¼ teaspoon black pepper

Directions:

- ❖ Spread a length of foil onto a work surface and place the salmon fillets in the middle.
- ❖ Blend olive oil, garlic, lime juice, parsley, and black pepper. Brush the mixture over the fillets. Fold the foil over and crimp the sides to make a packet.
- ❖ Place the packet into the slow cooker, cover, and cook on High for 2 hours
- ❖ Serve hot.

78) Delicious Puttanesca with Fresh Shrimp

Preparation Time: 5 minutes

Cooking Time: 15 minutes

Servings: 2

Nutrition: Calories 214, 10 g fat, 2 g fiber, 26 g protein

Ingredients:

- 2 tablespoons extra-virgin olive oil
- 3 anchovy fillets, drained and chopped
- 3 garlic cloves, minced
- ½ teaspoon crushed red pepper
- 1 (14.5-ounces) can low-sodium or no-salt-added diced tomatoes, undrained
- 1 (2.25-ounces) can sliced black olives, drained
- 2 tablespoons capers
- 1 tablespoon chopped fresh oregano
- 1-pound fresh raw shrimp, shells and tails removed

Directions:

❖ In a large skillet over medium heat, heat the oil. Mix in the anchovies, garlic, and crushed red pepper.

❖ Cook for 3 minutes, stirring frequently and mashing up the anchovies with a wooden spoon until they have melted into the oil.

❖ Stir in the tomatoes with their juices, olives, capers, and oregano. Turn up the heat to medium-high, and bring to a simmer.

❖ When the sauce is lightly bubbling, stir in the shrimp. Reduce the heat to medium, and cook the shrimp for 6 to 8 minutes, or until they turn pink and white, stirring occasionally, and serve.

79) Different Spicy Lasagna

Preparation Time: 15 minutes

Cooking Time: 40 minutes

Servings: 4

Nutrition: Calories: 194, Fat: 17.4g, Carbs:7g, Protein:7g

Ingredients:

- 2 tbsp butter
- 1 ½ lb ground tempeh
- Salt and ground black pepper to taste
- 1 tsp garlic powder
- 1 tsp onion powder
- 2 tbsp coconut flour
- 1 ½ cup grated mozzarella cheese
- 1/3 cup parmesan cheese
- 2 cups crumbled cottage cheese
- 1 large egg, beaten into a bowl
- 2 cups unsweetened marinara sauce
- 1 tbsp dried Italian mixed herbs
- ¼ tsp red chili flakes
- 4 large yellow squash, sliced
- ¼ cup fresh basil leaves

Directions:

❖ Preheat the oven to 375 F and grease a baking dish with cooking spray. Set aside.

❖ Melt the butter in a large skillet over medium heat and Cooking Time: the tempeh until brown, 10 minutes. Set aside to cool.

❖ In a medium bowl, mix the garlic powder, onion powder, coconut flour, black pepper, mozzarella cheese, half of the parmesan cheese, cottage cheese, and egg. Set aside.

❖ In another bowl, combine the marinara sauce, mixed herbs, and red chili flakes. Set aside.

❖ Make a single layer of the squash slices in the baking dish; spread a quarter of the egg mixture on top, a layer of the tempeh, then a quarter of the marinara sauce. Repeat the layering process in the same

❖ Ingredient proportions and sprinkle the top with the remaining parmesan cheese.

❖ Bake in the oven until golden brown on top, 30 minutes.

❖ Remove the dish from the oven, allow cooling for 5 minutes, garnish with the basil leaves, slice and serve.

80) Italian Green Seitan

Preparation Time: 15 minutes

Cooking Time: 18 minutes

Servings: 4

Nutrition: Calories: 582, Fat: 49.7g, Carbs:8g, Protein:31g,

Ingredients:

- 1 ½ lb seitan
- 3 tbsp almond flour
- Black pepper to taste
- 2 large zucchinis, cut into 2-inch slices
- 4 tbsp olive oil
- 2 tsp Italian mixed herb blend
- ½ cup vegetable broth

Directions:

❖ Preheat the oven to 400 F.

❖ Cut the seitan into strips and set aside.

❖ In a zipper bag, add the almond flour, salt, and black pepper. Mix and add the seitan slices. Seal the bag and shake to coat the seitan with the seasoning.

❖ Grease a baking sheet with cooking spray and arrange the zucchinis on the baking sheet. Season with black pepper, and drizzle with 2 tablespoons of olive oil.

❖ Using tongs, remove the seitan from the almond flour mixture, shake off the excess flour, and put two to three seitan strips on each zucchini.

❖ Season with the herb blend and drizzle again with olive oil.

❖ Cooking Time: in the oven for 8 minutes; remove the sheet and carefully pour in the vegetable broth. Bake further for 5 to 10 minutes or until the seitan cooks through.

❖ Remove from the oven and serve warm with low carb bread.

Chapter 6 -   Soup Recipes

81) Smoked Red Soup

Preparation Time: 10 minutes

Cooking Time: 17 minutes

Servings: 06

Nutrition: Calories 119 Fat 14 g Carbs 19 g Protein 5g

Ingredients:

- 1¼ cups red lentils, rinsed
- 4 cups of water
- ½ cup diced red bell pepper
- 1¼ cups red salsa
- 1 tablespoon chili powder
- 1 tablespoon dried oregano
- 1 teaspoon smoked paprika
- ¼ teaspoon black pepper
- ¾ cup frozen sweet corn
- 2 tablespoons lime juice

Directions:

- ❖ In a saucepan, add all the ingredients except the corn.
- ❖ Put on saucepan's lid and Cooking Time: for 15 minutes at a simmer.
- ❖ Stir in corn and Cooking Time: for another 2 minutes.
- ❖ Serve.

82) Lettuce Egg Soup Bowl

Preparation Time: 15 minutes

Cooking Time: 10 minutes

Servings: 2

Nutrition: Calories: 158 Carbs: 6.9g Fats: 7.3g Proteins: 15.4g

Ingredients:

- 32 oz vegetable broth
- 2 eggs
- 1 head romaine lettuce, chopped

Directions:

- ❖ Bring the vegetable broth to a boil and reduce the heat. Poach the eggs for 5 minutes in the broth and remove them into 2 bowls.
- ❖ Stir in romaine lettuce into the broth and cook for 4 minutes. Dish out in a bowl and serve hot.

83) Cayenne Kale and Mushrooms Soup

Preparation Time: 10 minutes

Cooking Time: 5 hrs. 5 minutes

Servings: 08

Nutrition: Calories 231 Fat 20.1 g Carbs 19,9 g Protein 4.6 g

Ingredients:

- ¼ cup olive oil
- 10 ounces button mushrooms, cleaned, and sliced
- 1½ teaspoons smoked paprika
- 1 pinch ground cayenne pepper
- 1 large onion, diced
- 2 cloves garlic, minced
- 2 pounds russet potatoes, peeled and diced
- 7 cups vegetable broth
- 8 ounces kale, sliced
- ½ teaspoon black pepper

Directions:

- ❖ In a pan, heat cooking oil and sauté mushrooms for 12 minutes.
- ❖ Season the mushrooms with salt, cayenne pepper, and paprika.
- ❖ Add olive oil and onion to a slow cooker.
- ❖ Sauté for 5 minutes then toss in rest of the soup ingredients.
- ❖ Put on the slow cooker's lid and Cooking Time: for 5 hours on low heat.
- ❖ Once done, puree the soup with a hand blender.
- ❖ Stir in sautéed mushrooms.
- ❖ Serve.

84) Coco Butternut Soup

Preparation Time: 15 minutes

Cooking Time: 1 hour & 35 minutes

Servings: 4

Nutrition: Calories: 149 Carbs: 6.6g Fats: 11.6g Proteins: 5.4g

Ingredients:

- 1 small onion, chopped
- 4 cups chicken broth
- 1 butternut squash
- 3 tablespoons coconut oil
- Nutmeg and pepper, to taste

Directions:

- ❖ Put oil and onions in a large pot and add onions. Sauté for about 3 minutes and add chicken broth and butternut squash.
- ❖ Simmer for about 1 hour on medium heat and transfer into an immersion blender. Pulse until smooth and season with pepper and nutmeg.
- ❖ Return to the pot and cook for about 30 minutes. Dish out and serve hot.

85) Cauliflower Broth with Leek

Preparation Time: 15 minutes

Cooking Time: 1 hour & 31 minutes

Servings: 4

Nutrition: Calories: 185 Carbs: 5.8g Fats: 12.7g Proteins: 10.8g

Ingredients:

- 4 cups chicken broth
- ½ cauliflower head, chopped
- 1 leek, chopped
- Black pepper, to taste

Directions:

- ❖ Put the cauliflower, leek and chicken broth into the pot and cook for about 1 hour on medium heat. Transfer into an immersion blender and pulse until smooth.
- ❖ Cook on for about 30 minutes on low heat. Season with pepper and serve.

86) Split Veggie Soup

Preparation Time: 10 minutes

Cooking Time: 6 hours

Servings: 12

Nutrition: Calories 361 Fat 16.3 g Carbs 29.3 g Protein 3.3 g

Ingredients:

- 1 cup dried, green split peas
- 2 cups celery, chopped
- 2 cups sliced carrots
- 1½ cups cauliflower, chopped
- 2 ounces dried shiitake mushrooms, chopped
- 9 ounces frozen artichoke hearts
- 11 cups water
- 1 teaspoon garlic powder
- 1½ teaspoon onion powder
- ½ teaspoon black pepper
- 1 tablespoon parsley
- ½ teaspoon ginger
- ½ teaspoon ground mustard seed
- ½ tablespoon brown rice vinegar

Directions:

- ❖ Add all the ingredients to a slow cooker.
- ❖ Put on the slow cooker's lid and Cooking
- ❖ Time: for 6 hours on low heat.
- ❖ Once done, garnish as desired.
- ❖ Serve warm.

87) Minestrone Bean Soup

Preparation Time: 10 minutes

Cooking Time: 2hrs 2 minutes

Servings: 4

Nutrition: Calories 205 Fat 19.7 g Carbs 26.1 g Protein 5.2 g

Ingredients:

- ½ sweet onion, chopped
- 4 garlic cloves, chopped
- 1 small head broccoli, chopped
- 2 stalks celery, chopped
- 1 cup green peas
- 3 green onions, chopped
- 2¾ cups vegetable broth
- 4 cups leafy greens
- 1 (15 ouncecan of cannellini beans
- Juice from 1 lemon
- 2 tablespoons fresh dill, chopped
- 5 fresh mint leaves
- ½ cup coconut milk
- Fresh herbs and peas, to garnish

Directions:

- ❖ In a slow cooker, add olive oil and onion.
- ❖ Sauté for 2 minutes then toss in the rest of the soup ingredients.
- ❖ Put on the slow cooker's lid and Cooking
- ❖ Time: for 2 hours on low heat.
- ❖ Once done, blend the soup with a hand blender.
- ❖ Garnish with fresh herbs and peas.
- ❖ Serve warm.

88) Swiss Coco Whisked Egg Soup

Preparation Time: 15 minutes

Cooking Time: 10 minutes

Servings: 4

Nutrition: Calories: 185 Carbs: 2.9g Fats: 11g Proteins: 18.3g

Ingredients:

- 3 cups bone broth
- 2 eggs, whisked
- 1 teaspoon ground oregano
- 3 tablespoons butter
- 2 cups Swiss chard, chopped
- 2 tablespoons coconut aminos
- 1 teaspoon ginger, grated
- Black pepper, to taste

Directions:

- ❖ Heat the bone broth in a saucepan and add whisked eggs while stirring slowly. Add the swiss chard, butter, coconut aminos, ginger, oregano and black pepper. Cook for about 10 minutes and serve hot.

89) Spinach and Mushroom Soup with Fresh Cream

Preparation Time: 15 minutes

Cooking Time: 10 minutes

Servings: 4

Nutrition: Calories: 160 Carbs: 7g Fats: 13.3g Proteins: 4.7g

Ingredients:

- 1 cup spinach, cleaned and chopped
- 100g mushrooms, chopped
- 1onion
- 6 garlic cloves
- ½ teaspoon red chili powder
- Black pepper, to taste
- 3 tablespoons buttermilk
- 1 teaspoon almond flour
- 2 cups chicken broth
- 3 tablespoons butter
- ¼ cup fresh cream for garnish

Directions:

- ❖ Heat butter in a pan and add onions and garlic. Sauté for about 3 minutes and add spinach and red chili powder.
- ❖ Sauté for about 4 minutes and add mushrooms. Transfer into a blender and blend to make a puree. Return to the pan and add buttermilk and almond flour for creamy texture.
- ❖ Mix well and simmer for about 2 minutes. Garnish with fresh cream and serve hot.

90) Veggie Soup with Peanut Butter

Preparation Time: 10 minutes

Cooking Time: 4 hrs. 5 minutes

Servings: 06

Nutrition: Calories 201 Fat 8.9 g Carbs 24.7 g Protein 15.3 g

Ingredients:

- 1 tablespoon water
- 6 cups sweet potatoes, peeled and chopped
- 2 cups onions, chopped
- 1 cup celery, chopped
- 4 large cloves garlic, chopped
- 2 teaspoons cumin seeds
- 3½ teaspoons ground coriander
- 1 teaspoon paprika
- ½ teaspoon crushed red pepper flakes
- 2 cups vegetable stock
- 3 cups water
- 4 tablespoons fresh ginger, grated
- 2 tablespoons natural peanut butter
- 2 cups cooked chickpeas
- 4 tablespoons lime juice
- Fresh cilantro, chopped
- Chopped peanuts, to garnish

Directions:

- ❖ In a slow cooker, add olive oil and onion.
- ❖ Sauté for 5 minutes then toss in the rest of the soup ingredients except chickpeas.
- ❖ Put on the slow cooker's lid and Cooking Time: for 4 hours on low heat.
- ❖ Once done, blend the soup with a hand blender.
- ❖ Stir in chickpeas and garnish with cilantro and peanuts.
- ❖ Serve warm.

91) Simple Red Lentil Soup

Preparation Time: 40 minutes

Cooking Time:

Servings: 3

Nutrition: Carbs: 15.3 g Protein: 6.2 g Fats: 0.3 g Calories: 90

Ingredients:

- Split red lentils: 1 cup
- Carrots: 1 cup grated
- Water: 6 cups
- Onion: 1 large coarsely chopped

Directions:

- ❖ Take a large saucepan and add water and bring to boil
- ❖ Add the chopped onions, carrots, lentils and bring to boil
- ❖ Lower the heat to medium and Cooking
- ❖ Time: for 20 minutes with partial cover
- ❖ Add the mixture to the high-speed blender to make a puree
- ❖ Whisk in water if desired
- ❖ Add again to the pan and slowly heat on a low flame for 10-15 minutes
- ❖ Add herbs or spices in between to augment the taste

92) Creamy Squash Soup

Preparation Time: 15 minutes

Cooking Time: 27 minutes

Servings: 5

Nutrition: Calories: 109 Carbs: 4.9g Fats: 8.5g Proteins: 3g

Ingredients:

- 1½ cups beef bone broth
- 1 small onion, peeled and grated.
- ¼ teaspoon poultry seasoning
- 2 small Delicata Squash, chopped
- 2 garlic cloves, minced
- 2 tablespoons olive oil
- ¼ teaspoon black pepper
- 1 small lemon, juiced
- 5 tablespoons sour cream

Directions:

- ❖ Put Delicata Squash and water in a medium pan and bring to a boil. Reduce the heat and cook for about 20 minutes. Drain and set aside.
- ❖ Put olive oil, onions, garlic and poultry seasoning in a small sauce pan. Cook for about 2 minutes and add broth. Allow it to simmer for 5 minutes and remove from heat.
- ❖ Whisk in the lemon juice and transfer the mixture in a blender. Pulse until smooth and top with sour cream.

93) Asparagus and Seed Soup with Cashew Cream

Preparation Time: 30 minutes

Cooking Time:

Servings: 2

Nutrition: Carbs: 11 g Protein: 9.4 g Fats: 18.3 g Calories: 243.5

Ingredients:

- Asparagus: 2 cups
- Vegetable stock: 4 cups
- Sesame seed: 2 tbsp
- Lemon juice: 1 tbsp
- Garlic: 4 cloves crushed
- Cashew cream: ½ cup
- Onion: 1 chopped
- Olive oil: 2 tbsp
- Pepper: as per your taste

Directions:

- ❖ Take a large saucepan and add olive oil to it
- ❖ Fry onion and garlic till it turns golden brown
- ❖ Chop asparagus and add to the pan along with the vegetable stock
- ❖ Let it boil and then Cooking Time: on low heat for 20 minutes
- ❖ When ready, add sesame seeds, lemon juice, and pepper as per your taste
- ❖ Serve with cashew cream on top

94) Spicy Bean Carrot and Lentil Soup

Preparation Time: 45 minutes

Cooking Time:

Servings: 4

Nutrition: Carbs: 425 g Protein: 8.17 g Fats: 4 g Calories: 148.75

Ingredients:

- Red lentils: 1 cup washed and drained
- Carrot: 2 medium chopped
- Beans: 1 cup drained
- Water: 3 cups
- Garlic: 3 cloves minced
- Onion: 1 medium finely chopped
- Ground cumin: 1 tsp
- Nutmeg: 1 tsp
- Ground coriander: 1 tsp
- Ground allspice: 1 tsp
- Ground cinnamon: 1 tsp
- Ground cayenne: ½ tsp
- Black pepper: as per your taste
- Extra virgin olive oil: 2 tbsp
- Cilantro: 1 tbsp chopped

Directions:

- ❖ Take a soup pot and heat oil in it on a medium flame
- ❖ Add onion and fry for 4-5 minutes
- ❖ Add carrot and garlic and stir for 5 minutes
- ❖ Wash lentils and add them to the pot
- ❖ Add water and bring to boil
- ❖ Lower the heat and Cooking Time: and cover for 15 minutes till lentil softens
- ❖ Add the remaining ingredients except for cilantro and Cooking Time: for an additional 15 minutes
- ❖ Serve warm with cilantro on top

95) Broccoli Ginger Soup with Herbs

Preparation Time: 15 minutes

Cooking Time: 37 minutes

Servings: 6

Nutrition: Calories: 183 Carbs: 5.2g Fats: 15.6g Proteins: 6.1g

Ingredients:

- 3 tablespoons ghee
- 5 garlic cloves
- 1 teaspoon sage
- ¼ teaspoon ginger
- 2 cups broccoli
- 1 small onion
- 1 teaspoon oregano
- ½ teaspoon parsley
- Black pepper, to taste
- 6 cups vegetable broth
- 4 tablespoons butter

Directions:

- ❖ Put ghee, onions, spices and garlic in a pot and cook for 3 minutes. Add broccoli and cook for about 4 minutes. Add vegetable broth, cover and allow it to simmer for about 30 minutes.
- ❖ Transfer into a blender and blend until smooth. Add the butter to give it a creamy delicious texture and flavor

96) Creamy Kabocha Soup

Preparation Time: 15 minutes

Cooking Time: 39 minutes

Servings: 8

Nutrition: Calories: 186 Carbs: 10.4g Fats: 14.9g Proteins: 3.7g

Ingredients:

- 1 apple, chopped
- 1 whole kabocha pumpkin, peeled, seeded and cubed
- 1 cup almond flour
- ¼ cup ghee
- 1 pinch cardamom powder
- 2 quarts water
- ¼ cup coconut cream
- 1 pinch ground black pepper

Directions:

- ❖ Heat ghee in the bottom of a heavy pot and add apples. Cook for about 5 minutes on a medium flame and add pumpkin.
- ❖ Sauté for about 3 minutes and add almond flour. Sauté for about 1 minute and add water. Lower the flame and cook for about 30 minutes.
- ❖ Transfer the soup into an immersion blender and blend until smooth. Top with coconut cream and serve.

97) Beans and Green Soup

Preparation Time: 20 minutes

Cooking Time:

Servings: 3

Nutrition: Carbs: 29.86 g Protein: 12.9 g Fats: 1.2 g Calories: 144

Ingredients:

- Cannellini beans: 1 cup rinsed and drained
- Artichoke hearts: 2 cups drained and chopped
- Frozen chopped spinach: 2 cups
- Water: 3 cups + 1 cup
- Garlic: 4 cloves chopped
- Onion: 1 medium chopped
- Italian herb blend: 2 tsp
- Black pepper: as per your taste

Directions:

- ❖ Take a blender and add onion, garlic, drained beans, herb blend, and pepper and add water
- ❖ Blend to give a smooth texture
- ❖ Add this puree to a large pan and Cooking Time: on medium-high heat
- ❖ When it initiates to boil, lower the heat and stir in between
- ❖ Let the mixture to thicken a bit
- ❖ Add one cup of water and spinach and blend
- ❖ Also, add artichokes and heat for 5 minutes
- ❖ Season with pepper if desired and serve

98) Sweety Onion Soup

Preparation Time: 15 minutes

Cooking Time: 335 minutes

Servings: 6

Nutrition: Calories: 198 Carbs: 6g Fats: 19.6g Proteins: 2.9g

Ingredients:
- 5 tablespoons butter
- 500 g brown onion medium
- 4 drops liquid stevia
- 4 tablespoons olive oil
- 3 cups beef stock

Directions:
- ❖ Put the butter and olive oil in a large pot over medium low heat and add onions. Cook for about 5 minutes and stir in stevia.
- ❖ Cook for another 5 minutes and add beef stock. Reduce the heat to low and simmer for about 25 minutes. Dish out into soup bowls and serve hot.

99) Lentils and Bean Mix in Masala Soup

Preparation Time: 40 minutes

Cooking Time:

Servings: 2

Nutrition: Carbs: 51.5 g Protein: 19.1 g Fats: 15.3 g Calories: 420

Ingredients:
- Red lentils: 1 cups
- Tomatoes: 1 cup can diced
- Beans: 1 cup can rinsed and drained
- Garam masala: 1 tbsp
- Vegetable oil: 2 tbsp
- Onion: 1 cup chopped
- Garlic: 3 cloves minced
- Ground cumin: 2 tbsp
- Smoked paprika: 1 tsp
- Celery: 1 cup chopped
- Lime juice and zest: 3 tbsp
- Fresh cilantro: 3 tbsp chopped
- Water: 2 cups

Directions:
- ❖ Take a large pot and add oil to it
- ❖ On the medium flame, add garlic, celery and onion
- ❖ Add garam masala, and cumin to them and stir for 5 minutes till they turn brown
- ❖ Add water, lentils, and tomatoes with the juice and bring to boil
- ❖ Bring to boil and heat for 25-30 minutes on low flame
- ❖ Add in lime juice and zest and beans of your choice and stir
- ❖ Serve with cilantro on top

100) Cauli Soup with Matcha Tea

Preparation Time: 15 minutes

Cooking Time: 13 minutes

Servings: 6

Nutrition: Calories: 79 Carbs: 3.8g Fats: 7.1g Proteins: 1.3g

Ingredients:
- 2 teaspoons thyme powder
- 1 head cauliflower
- 3 cups vegetable stock
- ½ teaspoon matcha green tea powder
- 3 tablespoons olive oil
- Black pepper, to taste
- 5 garlic cloves, chopped

Directions:
- ❖ Put the vegetable stock, thyme and matcha powder to a large pot over medium-high heat and bring to a boil. Add cauliflower and cook for about 10 minutes.
- ❖ Meanwhile, put the olive oil and garlic in a small sauce pan and cook for about 1 minute. Add the garlic and black pepper and cook for about 2 minutes.
- ❖ Transfer into an immersion blender and blend until smooth. Dish out and serve immediately.

Chapter 7 -   Snack Recipe

101) Smoked Thaini Beets Hummus

Preparation Time: 10 minutes

Cooking Time: 60 minutes

Servings: 4

Nutrition: Calories: 50.1 Cal Fat: 2.5 g Carbs: 5 g Protein: 2 g

Ingredients:
- 15 ounces cooked chickpeas
- 3 small beets
- 1 teaspoon minced garlic
- 1/2 teaspoon smoked paprika
- 1/4 teaspoon red chili flakes
- 2 tablespoons olive oil
- 1 lemon, juiced
- 2 tablespoon tahini
- 1 tablespoon chopped almonds
- 1 tablespoon chopped cilantro

Directions:
- ❖ Drizzle oil over beets, then wrap beets in a foil and bake for 60 minutes at 425 degrees F until tender.
- ❖ When done, let beet cool for 10 minutes, then peel and dice them and place them in a food processor.
- ❖ Add remaining ingredients and pulse for 2 minutes until smooth, tip the hummus in a bowl, drizzle with some more oil, and then serve straight away.

102) Lemony Fava Cream

Preparation Time: 10 minutes

Cooking Time: 30 minutes

Servings: 4

Nutrition: Calories 405 Fat 1 g Carbs 75 g Protein 25 g

Ingredients:
- 2 cups Santorini fava (yellow split peas), rinsed
- 2 medium onions, chopped
- 2 ½ cups water
- 2 cups +2 tablespoons vegetable broth
- To garnish:
- Lemon juice as required
- Chopped parsley

Directions:
- ❖ Place fava in a large pot. Add onions, broth, water and stir. Place over medium heat. When it begins to boil, reduce the heat and cook until fava is tender.
- ❖ Remove from heat and cool. Blend until creamy. Ladle into small plates. Add lemon juice and stir. Garnish with parsley and serve.

103) Zucchini Hummus with Cumin

Preparation Time: 5 minutes

Cooking Time: 0 minute

Servings: 8

Nutrition: Calories: 65 Cal Fat: 5 g Carbs: 3 g Protein: 2 g

Ingredients:
- 1 cup diced zucchini
- 1 teaspoon minced garlic
- 2 teaspoons ground cumin
- 3 tablespoons lemon juice
- 1/3 cup tahini

Directions:
- ❖ Place all the ingredients in a food processor and pulse for 2 minutes until smooth.
- ❖ Tip the hummus in a bowl, drizzle with oil and serve.

104) Crispy Hummus Bell Pepper

Preparation Time: 10 minutes

Cooking Time: 0 minutes

Servings: 2

Nutrition: Calories 136 Fat 7 g Carbs 13 g Protein 6 g

Ingredients:
- 4 tablespoons hummus
- 2 large whole grain crisp bread
- 4 tablespoons crumbled feta
- 1 small bell pepper, diced

Directions:
- ❖ Top the pieces of crisp bread with hummus. Sprinkle feta cheese and bell peppers and serve.

105) Totopos Enchilados

Preparation Time: 10 minutes

Cooking Time: 15 minutes

Servings: 4

Nutrition: Calories: 150 Fat: 7 g Carbs: 18 g Protein: 2 g

Ingredients:
- 12 ounces whole-wheat tortillas
- 4 tablespoons chipotle seasoning
- 1 tablespoon olive oil
- 4 limes, juiced

Directions:
- ❖ Whisk together oil and lime juice, brush it well on tortillas, then sprinkle with chipotle seasoning and bake for 15 minutes at 350 degrees F until crispy, turning halfway.
- ❖ When done, let the tortilla cool for 10 minutes, then break it into chips and serve.

106) Garlic Tomato Italian Toast

Preparation Time: 10 minutes

Cooking Time: 10 minutes

Servings: 3

Nutrition: Calories 162 Fat 4 g Carbs 29 g Protein 4 g

Ingredients:
- 3 tomatoes, finely chopped
- 1 clove garlic, minced
- ¼ teaspoon garlic powder (optional)
- A handful basil leaves, coarsely chopped
- Pepper to taste
- ½ teaspoon olive oil
- ½ tablespoon balsamic vinegar
- ½ tablespoon butter
- ½ baguette French bread or Italian bread, cut into ½ inch thick slices

Directions:
- ❖ Add tomatoes, garlic and basil in a bowl and toss well. Add pepper. Drizzle oil and vinegar and toss well. Set aside for an hour.
- ❖ Melt the butter and brush it over the baguette slices. Place in an oven and toast the slices. Sprinkle the tomato mixture on top and serve right away.

107) Spanish Potato Tortillas

Preparation Time: 10 minutes

Cooking Time: 8 minutes

Servings: 10

Nutrition: Calories: 70 Fat: 3 g Carbs: 8 g Protein: 1 g

Ingredients:
- 1/3 cup quinoa flour
- 1½ cups shredded sweet potato
- 1 cup grated carrot
- 1/3 teaspoon ground black pepper
- 2 teaspoons curry powder
- 2 flax eggs
- 2 tablespoons coconut oil

Directions:
- ❖ Place all the ingredients in a bowl, except for oil, stir well until combined and then shape the mixture into ten small patties
- ❖ Take a large pan, place it over medium-high heat, add oil and when it melts, add patties in it and Cooking Time: for 3 minutes per side until browned.
- ❖ Serve straight away

108) Turkish Delicious Spiced Falafel

Preparation Time: 30 minutes

Cooking Time: 15 minutes

Servings: 2

Nutrition: Calories 93 Fat 3.8 g Carbs 1.3 g Protein 3.9 g

Ingredients:
- 1 cup dried chickpeas (do not use cooked or canned)
- ½ cup fresh parsley leaves, discard stems
- ¼ cup fresh dill leaves, discard stems
- ½ cup fresh cilantro leaves
- 4 cloves garlic, peeled
- ½ tablespoon ground black pepper
- ½ tablespoon ground coriander
- ½ tablespoon ground cumin
- ½ teaspoon cayenne pepper (optional)
- ½ teaspoon baking powder
- ¼ teaspoon baking soda
- 1 tablespoon toasted sesame seeds
- Oil, as required

Directions:
- ❖ Rinse chickpeas and soak in water overnight. Cover with at least 3 inches of water. Drain and dry by patting with a kitchen towel.
- ❖ Add all the fresh herbs into a food processor. Process until finely chopped. Add chickpeas, spices and garlic and pulse for not more than 40 seconds each time until smooth.
- ❖ Transfer into a container. Cover and chill for at least 1 hour or until use. Divide the mixture into 12 equal portions and shape into patties.
- ❖ Place a deep pan over medium heat. Pour enough oil to cover at least 3 inches from the bottom of the pan.
- ❖ When the oil is well heated, but not smoking, drop falafel, a few at a time and fry until medium brown.
- ❖ Remove with a spoon and place on a plate lined with paper towels. Serve with a dip of your choice.

109) Red Pesto Bruschetta

Preparation Time: 5 minutes

Cooking Time: 0 minute

Servings: 4

Nutrition: Calories: 214 Fat: 7.2 g Carbs: 32 g Protein: 6.5 g

Ingredients:
- 1 small tomato, sliced
- ¼ teaspoon ground black pepper
- 1 tablespoon vegan pesto
- 2 tablespoons hummus
- 1 slice of whole-grain bread, toasted
- Hemp seeds as needed for garnishing

Directions:
- ❖ Spread hummus on one side of the toast, top with tomato slices and then drizzle with pesto.
- ❖ Sprinkle black pepper on the toast along with hemp seeds and then serve straight away.

110) _Cheesy Low-Fat Yogurt Dip_

Preparation Time: 15 minutes + chilling

Cooking Time: 0 minutes

Servings: 8 (2 tablespoons dip without vegetable sticks)

Nutrition: Calories 68 Fat 4 g Carbs 5 g Protein 4 g

Ingredients:

- 2 cups plain low-fat yogurt
- ¼ cup crumbled feta cheese
- 3 tablespoons chopped walnuts or pine nuts
- 1 teaspoon chopped fresh oregano or marjoram or ½ teaspoon dried oregano or marjoram, crushed
- Freshly ground pepper to taste
- 1 tablespoon snipped dried tomatoes (not oil packed)
- Walnut halves to garnish
- Assorted vegetable sticks to serve

Directions:

- ❖ For yogurt dip, place 3 layers of cotton cheesecloth over a strainer. Place strainer over a bowl. Add yogurt into the strainer. Cover the strainer with cling wrap. Refrigerate for 24-48 hours.
- ❖ Discard the strained liquid and add yogurt into a bowl. Add feta cheese, walnuts, seasoning, and herbs and mix well. Cover and chill for an hour.
- ❖ Garnish with walnut halves. Serve with vegetable sticks.

111) _Exotic Hummus And Sprout Toast_

Preparation Time: 5 minutes

Cooking Time: 0 minute

Servings: 4

Nutrition: Calories: 200 Fat: 10.5 g Carbs: 22 g Protein: 7 g

Ingredients:

- 1/2 of a medium avocado, sliced
- 1 slice of whole-grain bread, toasted
- 2 tablespoons sprouts
- 2 tablespoons hummus
- ¼ teaspoon lemon zest
- ½ teaspoon hemp seeds
- ¼ teaspoon red pepper flakes

Directions:

- ❖ Spread hummus on one side of the toast and then top with avocado slices and sprouts.
- ❖ Sprinkle with lemon zest, hemp seeds, and red pepper flakes and then serve straight away.

112) _Rich Ricotta Snack_

Preparation Time: 5 minutes

Cooking Time: 0 minutes

Servings: 2

Nutrition: Calories 178 Fat 9 g Carbs 15 g Protein 11 g

Ingredients:

- 2/3 cup part-skim ricotta
- 2 clementine's, peeled, separated into segments, deseeded
- 4 teaspoons chopped pistachio nuts

Directions:

- ❖ Place 1/3 cup ricotta in each of 2 bowls. Divide the clementine segments equally and place over the ricotta. Sprinkle pistachio nuts on top and serve.

113) _Sweety Apple Toast with Cinnamon_

Preparation Time: 5 minutes

Cooking Time: 0 minute

Servings: 4

Nutrition: Calories: 212 Fat: 7 g Carbs: 35 g Protein: 4 g

Ingredients:

- ½ of a small apple, cored, sliced
- 1 slice of whole-grain bread, toasted
- 1 tablespoon honey
- 2 tablespoons hummus
- 1/8 teaspoon cinnamon

Directions:

- ❖ Spread hummus on one side of the toast, top with apple slices and then drizzle with honey.
- ❖ Sprinkle cinnamon on it and then serve straight away.

114) _Crispy Zucchini_

Preparation Time: 10 minutes

Cooking Time: 120 minutes

Servings: 4

Nutrition: Calories: 54 Fat: 5 g Carbs: 1 g Protein: 6 g

Ingredients:

- 1 large zucchini, thinly sliced
- 2 tablespoons olive oil

Directions:

- ❖ Pat dry zucchini slices and then spread them in an even layer on a baking sheet lined with parchment sheet.
- ❖ Add oil, brush this mixture over zucchini slices on both sides and then bake for 2 hours or more until brown and crispy.
- ❖ When done, let the chips cool for 10 minutes and then serve straight away.

115) _Summer Vegetarian Wraps_

Preparation Time: 15 minutes

Cooking Time: 10 minutes

Servings: 2

Nutrition: Calories: 262; Fat: 15g; Carbs: 23g; Protein: 7g

Ingredients:
- 1½ cups seedless cucumber, peeled and chopped (about 1 large cucumber)
- 1 cup chopped tomato (about 1 large tomato)
- ½ cup finely chopped fresh mint
- 1 (2.25-ounce) can sliced black olives (about ½ cup), drained
- ¼ cup diced red onion (about ¼ onion)
- 2 tablespoons extra-virgin olive oil
- 1 tablespoon red wine vinegar
- ¼ teaspoon freshly ground black pepper
- ½ cup crumbled goat cheese (about 2 ounces)
- 4 whole-wheat flatbread wraps or soft whole-wheat tortillas

Directions:
- In a large bowl, mix together the cucumber, tomato, mint, olives, and onion until well combined.
- In a small bowl, whisk together the oil, vinegar, and pepper. Drizzle the dressing over the salad, and mix gently.
- With a knife, spread the goat cheese evenly over the four wraps. Spoon a quarter of the salad filling down the middle of each wrap.
- Fold up each wrap: Start by folding up the bottom, then fold one side over and fold the other side over the top. Repeat with the remaining wraps and serve.

116) _Spiced Pineapple Mix_

Preparation Time: 15 minutes

Cooking Time: 90 minutes

Servings: 4

Nutrition: Calories: 230 Fat: 17.5 g Carbs: 11.5 g Protein: 6.5 g

Ingredients:
- 5 cups mixed nuts
- 1 cup chopped dried pineapple
- 1 cup pumpkin seed
- 1 teaspoon garlic powder
- 1 teaspoon onion powder
- 2 teaspoons paprika
- 1/4 cup coconut sugar
- 1/2 teaspoon red chili powder
- 1/2 teaspoon ground black pepper
- 1 tablespoon red pepper flakes
- 1/2 tablespoon red curry powder
- 2 tablespoons soy sauce
- 2 tablespoons coconut oil

Directions:
- Switch on the slow cooker, add all the ingredients in it except for dried pineapple and red pepper flakes, stir until combined and Cooking Time: for 90 minutes at high heat setting, stirring every 30 minutes.
- When done, spread the nut mixture on a baking sheet lined with parchment paper and let it cool.
- Then spread dried pineapple on top, sprinkle with red pepper flakes and serve.

117) _Salmon Wraps with Balsamic Vinegar_

Preparation Time: 20 minutes

Cooking Time: 60 minutes

Servings: 2

Nutrition: Calories: 336; Total Fat: 16g; Carbs: 23g; Protein: 32g

Ingredients:
- 1-pound salmon filet, cooked and flaked, or 3 (5-ounce) cans salmon
- ½ cup diced carrots (about 1 carrot)
- ½ cup diced celery (about 1 celery stalk)
- 3 tablespoons chopped fresh dill
- 3 tablespoons diced red onion (a little less than 1/8 onion)
- 2 tablespoons capers
- 1½ tablespoons extra-virgin olive oil
- 1 tablespoon aged balsamic vinegar
- ½ teaspoon freshly ground black pepper
- 4 whole-wheat flatbread wraps or soft whole-wheat tortillas

Directions:
- In a large bowl, mix together the salmon, carrots, celery, dill, red onion, capers, oil, vinegar and pepper.
- Divide the salmon salad among the flatbreads. Fold up the bottom of the flatbread, then roll up the wrap and serve.

118) _Incredible Dried Snack_

Preparation Time: 10 minutes

Cooking Time: 17 minutes

Servings: 2

Nutrition: 44g Carbs, 7g Fat, 13g Protein, 285 Calories 65

Ingredients:
- 3 c. water
- ¼ c. cashew nut
- 8 dried apricots
- 4 dried figs
- 1 tsp. cinnamon

Directions:
- In a pot, mix water and quinoa and
- Let simmer for 15 minutes, until the water evaporates.
- Chop dried fruit.
- When quinoa is cooked, stir in all other ingredients.
- Serve cold. Add milk, if desired.

119) *Crispy Beet with Rosemary*

Preparation Time: 10 minutes

Cooking Time: 20 minutes

Servings: 3

Nutrition: Calories: 79 Fat: 4.7 g Carbs: 8.6 g Protein: 1.5 g

Ingredients:

- 3 large beets, scrubbed, thinly sliced
- 1/8 teaspoon ground black pepper
- 3 sprigs of rosemary, leaves chopped
- 4 tablespoons olive oil

Directions:

- ❖ Spread beet slices in a single layer between two large baking sheets, brush the slices with oil, then season with spices and rosemary, toss until well coated, and bake for 20 minutes at 375 degrees F until crispy, turning halfway.
- ❖ When done, let the chips cool for 10 minutes and then serve.

120) *Sweety Oats with Cinnamon*

Preparation Time: 10 minutes

Cooking Time: 15 minutes

Servings: 2

Nutrition: Calories: 232, Fat: 5.7 g, Carbs: 48.1 g, Protein: 5.2 g

Ingredients:

- ½ tsp. cinnamon
- ¼ tsp. ginger
- 2 apples make half-inch chunks
- ½ c. oats, steel cut
- 1½ c. water
- Maple syrup
- Clove
- ¼ tsp. nutmeg

Directions:

- ❖ Take Instant Pot and careful y arrange it over a clean, dry kitchen platform.
- ❖ Turn on the appliance.
- ❖ In the cooking pot area, add the water, oats, cinnamon, ginger, clove, nutmeg and apple. Stir the ingredients gently.
- ❖ Close the pot lid and seal the valve to avoid any leakage. Find and press the "Manual" cooking setting and set cooking time to 5 minutes.
- ❖ Allow the recipe ingredients to cook for the set time, and after that, the timer reads "zero."
- ❖ Press "Cancel" and press "NPR" setting for natural pressure release. It takes 8-10 times for all inside pressure to release.
- ❖ Open the pot and arrange the cooked recipe in serving plates.
- ❖ Sweeten as needed with maple or agave syrup and serve immediately.
- ❖ Top with some chopped nuts, optional.

Chapter 8 -   Dessert and Smoothie Recipes

121) Cocoflakes Cantaloupe Yogurt with Raspberry

Preparation Time: 15 minutes

Cooking Time: 0 minutes

Servings: 6

Nutrition: Calories: 75 Fat: 4.1g Protein: 1.2g Carbs: 10.9g

Ingredients:

- 2 cups fresh raspberries, mashed
- 1 cup plain coconut yogurt
- ½ teaspoon vanilla extract
- 1 cantaloupe, peeled and sliced
- ½ cup toasted coconut flakes

Directions:

- Combine the mashed raspberries with yogurt and vanilla extract in a small bowl. Stir to mix well.
- Place the cantaloupe slices on a platter, then top with raspberry mixture and spread with toasted coconut. Serve immediately.

122) Plant-Based Berry and Banana Smoothie

Preparation Time: 5 minutes

Cooking Time:

Servings: 2

Nutrition: Calories 269, Fat 12.3g, Carbs 37.6g, Protein 6.4g

Ingredients:

- 2 cups, plant-based Milk
- 2 cups, Frozen or fresh berries
- ½ cup Frozen ripe bananas
- 2 teaspoons, Flax Seeds
- ¼ tsp, Vanilla
- ¼ tsp, Cinnamon

Directions:

- Mix together milk, flax seeds, and fruit. Blend in a high-power blender.
- Add cinnamon and vanilla. Blend until smooth.
- Serve and enjoy!

123) Delicious Apple Compote with Cinnamon

Preparation Time: 15 minutes

Cooking Time: 10 minutes

Servings: 4

Nutrition: Calories: 246 Fat: 0.9g Protein: 1.2g Carbs: 66.3g

Ingredients:

- 6 apples, peeled, cored, and chopped
- ¼ cup raw honey
- 1 teaspoon ground cinnamon
- ¼ cup apple juice

Directions:

- Put all the ingredients in a stockpot. Stir to mix well, then cook over medium-high heat for 10 minutes or until the apples are glazed by honey and lightly saucy. Stir constantly. Serve immediately.

124) Carrot and Prunes Smoothie with Walnuts

Preparation Time: 5 minutes

Cooking Time:

Servings: 4

Nutrition: Carbs: 14.9 g Protein: 3 g Fats: 4.5 g Calories: 103

Ingredients:

- Almond milk: 2 cups
- Prunes: 60 g
- Banana: 1
- Carrots: 150 g
- Walnuts: 30 g
- Ground cinnamon: ½ tsp
- Vanilla extract: 1 tsp

Directions:

- Add all the ingredients to the blender
- Blend on high speed to make it smooth

125) Choco Bombs

Preparation Time: 45 minutes

Cooking Time: 0 minutes

Servings: 15 balls

Nutrition: Calories: 146 Fat: 8.1g Protein: 4.2g Carbs: 16.9g

Ingredients:

- ¾ cup creamy peanut butter
- ¼ cup unsweetened cocoa powder
- 2 tablespoons softened almond butter
- ½ teaspoon vanilla extract
- 1¾ cups maple sugar

Directions:

- Line a baking sheet with parchment paper. Combine all the ingredients in a bowl. Stir to mix well.
- Divide the mixture into 15 parts and shape each part into a 1-inch ball. Arrange the balls on the baking sheet and refrigerate for at least 30 minutes, then serve chilled.

126) Dark Date and Banana Drink

Preparation Time: 5 minutes

Cooking Time:

Servings: 2

Nutrition: Carbs: 72.1 g Protein: 8 g Fats: 12.7 g Calories: 385

Ingredients:

- Unsweetened cocoa powder: 2 tbsp
- Unsweetened nut milk: 2 cups
- Almond butter: 2 tbsp
- Dried dates: 4 pitted
- Frozen bananas: 2 medium
- Ground cinnamon: ¼ tsp

Directions:

- Add all the ingredients to the blender
- Blend to form a smooth consistency

127) Sweety Watermelon Iced Flakes

Preparation Time: 10 minutes + 3 hours to freeze

Cooking Time: 0 minutes

Servings: 4

Nutrition: Calories: 153 Carbs: 39g Protein: 2g Fat: 1g

Ingredients:
- 4 cups watermelon cubes
- ¼ cup honey
- ¼ cup freshly squeezed lemon juice

Directions:
- ❖ In a blender, combine the watermelon, honey, and lemon juice. Purée all the ingredients, then pour into a 9-by-9-by-2-inch baking pan and place in the freezer.
- ❖ Every 30 to 60 minutes, run a fork across the frozen surface to fluff and create ice flakes. Freeze for about 3 hours total and serve.

128) Cashew and Fruit Mix Smoothie

Preparation Time: 5 minutes

Cooking Time:

Servings: 4

Nutrition: Carbs: 32.9 g Protein: 9.7 g Fats: 15 g Calories: 320

Ingredients:
- Pistachios: 1 cup
- Raw pumpkin: 175 g
- Cloves: 1
- Nutmeg: 1/8 tsp
- Dates: 4
- Banana: 1
- Ground ginger: 1/8 tsp
- Ground cinnamon: 1 tsp
- Cashew milk: 500 ml
- Ice: as per your need

Directions:
- ❖ Add all the ingredients to the blender
- ❖ Blend on high speed to make it smooth

129) Seed Butter Cookies

Preparation Time: 10 minutes

Cooking Time: 15 minutes

Servings: 14-16

Nutrition: Calories 218 Fat 12g Carbs 25g Protein 4g

Ingredients:
- 1 cup sesame seeds, hulled
- 1 cup sugar
- 8 tablespoons unsalted butter, softened
- 2 large eggs
- 1¼ cups flour

Directions:
- ❖ Preheat the oven to 350°F. Toast the sesame seeds on a baking sheet for 3 minutes. Set aside and let cool.
- ❖ Using a mixer, cream together the sugar and butter. Put the eggs one at a time until well-blended. Add the flour and toasted sesame seeds and mix until well-blended.
- ❖ Drop spoonful of cookie dough onto a baking sheet and form them into round balls, about 1-inch in diameter, similar to a walnut.
- ❖ Put in the oven and bake for 5 to 7 minutes or until golden brown. Let the cookies cool and enjoy.

130) Persimmon Healthy Smoothie

Preparation Time: 5 minutes

Cooking Time:

Servings: 1

Nutrition: Carbs: 37.1 g Protein: 6.5 g Fats: 5.4 g Calories: 183

Ingredients:
- Persimmon: 1
- Spinach: 1 cup
- Orange: 1
- Water: 1 cup
- Chia seeds: 1 tbsp

Directions:
- ❖ Add all the ingredients to the blender
- ❖ Blend to form a smooth consistency
- ❖ Add ice cubes from the top to chill it

131) Sweety Rice with Rose Water and Dried Figs

Preparation Time: 45 minutes

Cooking Time: 0 minutes

Servings: 2

Nutrition: Calories: 228; Fat: 6.1g; Carbs: 35.1g; Protein: 7.1g

Ingredients:
- 3 cups milk
- 1 cup water
- 2 tablespoons sugar
- 1/3 cup white rice, rinsed
- 1 tablespoon honey
- 4 dried figs, chopped
- 1/2 teaspoon cinnamon
- 1/2 teaspoon rose water

Directions:
- ❖ In a deep saucepan, bring the milk, water and sugar to a boil until the sugar has dissolved.
- ❖ Stir in the rice, honey, figs, raisins, cinnamon, and turn the heat to a simmer; let it simmer for about 40 minutes, stirring periodically to prevent your pudding from sticking.
- ❖ Afterwards, stir in the rose water. Divide the pudding between individual bowls and serve. Bon appétit!

132) _Fresh and Dry Smoothie_

Preparation Time: 5 minutes

Cooking Time:

Servings: 1

Nutrition: Carbs: 66.0 g Protein: 16.1 g Fats: 18 g Calories: 435

Ingredients:
- Fresh figs: 2
- Almond milk: 1 cup
- Dried date: 1 pitted
- Vanilla extract: ¼ tsp
- Sesame seeds: 2 tbsp

Directions:
- ❖ Add all the ingredients to the blender
- ❖ Blend to form a smooth consistency

133) _Greek Yogurt with Honey and Fruit Mix_

Preparation Time: 10 minutes

Cooking Time: 0 minutes

Servings: 2

Nutrition: Calories: 98; Fat: 0.2g; Carbs: 20.7g; Protein: 2.8g

Ingredients:
- 8 clementine orange segments
- 8 medium-sized strawberries
- 8 pineapple cubes
- 8 seedless grapes
- 1/2 cup Greek-style yogurt
- 1/2 teaspoon vanilla extract
- 2 tablespoons honey

Directions:
- ❖ Thread the fruits onto 4 skewers.
- ❖ In a mixing dish, thoroughly combine the yogurt, vanilla, and honey.
- ❖ Serve alongside your fruit kabobs for dipping. Bon appétit!

134) _Almond Berries and Banana Smoothie_

Preparation Time: 5 minutes

Cooking Time:

Servings: 2

Nutrition: Carbs: 14.9 g Protein: 2.2 g Fats: 1.6 g Calories: 92

Ingredients:
- Banana: 1 ripe
- Frozen berries: 200g
- Almond milk: 250ml

Directions:
- ❖ Add all the ingredients in the blender
- ❖ Blend to give a smooth consistency
- ❖ Pour to the glasses and serve

135) _Choco Walnuts Cube with Thaini_

Preparation Time: 10 minutes

Cooking Time: 0 minutes

Servings: 2

Nutrition: Calories: 198; Fat: 13g; Carbs: 17.3g; Protein: 4.6g

Ingredients:
- 8 ounces bittersweet chocolate
- 1 cup tahini paste
- 1/4 cup almonds, chopped
- 1/4 cup walnuts, chopped

Directions:
- ❖ Microwave the chocolate for about 30 seconds or until melted. Stir in the tahini, almonds, and walnuts.
- ❖ Spread the batter into a parchment-lined baking pan. Place in your refrigerator until set, for about 3 hours.
- ❖ Cut into cubes and serve well-chilled.

136) _Fruit Explosion Smoothie_

Preparation Time: 5 minutes

Cooking Time:

Servings: 2

Nutrition: Carbs: 52.8 g Protein: 6.4 g Fats: 19.5 g Calories: 407

Ingredients:
- Banana: 1 ripe sliced
- Almond milk: 1 cup
- Coconut oil: 1 tbsp
- Powdered ginger: 1 tsp
- Frozen fruit medley: 1 cup
- Chia seeds: 2 tbsp

Directions:
- ❖ Add all the ingredients in the blender
- ❖ Blend to give a smooth consistency
- ❖ Pour to the glasses and serve

137) _Greek Granola Berries_

Preparation Time: 10 minutes

Cooking Time: 0 minutes

Servings: 2

Nutrition: Calories: 238; Fat: 16.7g; Carbs: 53g; Protein: 21.6g

Ingredients:
- 2 cups Greek yogurt
- 2 cups mixed berries
- 1/2 cup granola

Directions:
- ❖ Alternate layers of mixed berries, granola, and yogurt until two dessert bowls are filled completely.
- ❖ Cover and place in your refrigerator until you're ready to serve. Bon appétit!

138) *Energy Almond Smoothie*

Preparation Time: 5 minutes

Cooking Time:

Servings: 1

Nutrition: Carbs: 41.2 g Protein: 8.9 g Fats: 3.9 g Calories: 220

Ingredients:

- Large banana: 1 frozen
- Fresh spinach: 1 cup
- Rolled oats: 2 tbsp
- Unsweetened almond milk: ¾ cup

Directions:

- ❖ Add all the ingredients to the blender
- ❖ Blend to form a smooth consistency

139) *Figs and Walnuts with Honey Topping*

Preparation Time: 20 Minutes

Cooking Time: 0 Minutes

Servings: 4

Nutrition: Calories: 110 Carbs: 26 Fat: 3g, Protein: 1g

Ingredients:

- 12 dried figs
- 2 Tbsps. thyme honey
- 2 Tbsps. sesame seeds
- 24 walnut halves

Directions:

- ❖ Cut off the tough stalk ends of the figs.
- ❖ Slice open each fig.
- ❖ Stuff the fig openings with two walnut halves and close
- ❖ Arrange the figs on a plate, drizzle with honey, and sprinkle the sesame seeds on it.
- ❖ Serve.

140) *Thaini Figs Smoothie*

Preparation Time: 5 minutes

Cooking Time:

Servings: 1

Nutrition: Carbs: 66.0 g

Protein: 12.1 g Fats: 16.5g Calories: 435

Ingredients:

- Dried date: 1 pitted
- Tahini: 1 tbsp
- Fresh figs: 2
- Almond milk: 1 cup
- Vanilla extract: ¼ tsp

Directions:

- ❖ Add all the ingredients to the blender
- ❖ Blend to form a smooth consistency

Chapter 9 - Simple Dr. Cole's Meal Plan – For Women

Day 1

3) Golden Coco Mix | Calories 259

21) Pasta with Delicious Spanish Salsa | Calories 364

62) Smoked Baby Spinach Stew | Calories 369

41) Veggie ChimiSalad | Calories 231

123) Delicious Apple Compote with Cinnamon | Calories 246

Total Calories: 1469

Day 2

10) Black Olives and Feta Bread | Calories 251

25) Chickpeas Tomato Pasta with Tamari | Calories 442

65) Veggie Ragù Noodles | Calories 353

46) Easy Creamy Kernel | Calories 306

125) Choco Bombs | Calories 146

Total Calories: 1498

Day 3

13) Vegetables Wraps with Soy Sauce | Calories 284

29) Spiced Kidney Pasta with Cilantro | Calories 274

67) Red Quinoa Burgers with Thaini Guacamole | Calories 343

48) Old School Panzanella | Calories 294

128) Cashew and Fruit Mix Smoothie | Calories 320

Total Calories: 1515

Day 4

19) Awesome Breakfast Muesli | Calories 250

31 Red Lentils Spaghetti with Herbs | Calories 335

72) Cold Spinach with Fruit Mix | Calories 296

53) Double Green Juicy Salad | Calories 237

140) Thaini Figs Smoothie | Calories 435

Total Calories: 1553

Day 5

7) Button Mushroom Omelette | Calories 189

35) Macaroni with Cherry and Peas | Calories 320

76) Hummus Quinoa with Edamame Bowl | Calories 381

56) Cheesy Asparagus Pesto Salad | Calories 220

138) Energy Almond Smoothie | Calories 220

Total Calories: 1330

Day 6

4) Delicious Agave Rice | Calories 192

37) Golden Rice with Pistachios | Calories 320

75) Cheesy Gnocchi with Shrimp | Calories 227

55) Asian Goji Salad | Calories 203

136) Fruit Explosion Smoothie | Calories 407

Total Calories: 1349

Day 7

2) Apple Warm Oatmeal | Calories 200

40) Bean Balls with Red pepper and Marinara Sauce | Calories 351

63) Green Chilis Chicken Breast | Calories 237

44) Noodles Salad with Peanut Butter Cream | Calories 361

126) Dark Date and Banana Drink | Calories 385

Total Calories: 1534

DASH

Diet Cookbook

On a Budget

Easy Dr. Cole's Diet Plan | Delicious and Budget Friendly Low Sodium Recipes to Lower Blood Pressure and Kickstart your Healthy Path

By Janeth Cole

Chapter 1 - Introduction

There are some essential things in today's life such as maintaining good health, which will allow us to enjoy life and have a budget according to our personal goals. In this introduction I will tell you what the DASH diet is and how to use it to your advantage in order to have a healthy budget and a healthy life.

What is the dash diet?

The Dietary Approaches to Stop Hypertension or DASH diet is a diet that favors a balanced intake of different major nutrients and a low sodium intake. It originally emerged from studies for the treatment of arterial hypertension, but it has been found to have multiple benefits. It basically consists of increasing the consumption of fruits, vegetables, fish, lean meat, low-fat dairy products, whole grains, seeds, nuts and legumes. Avoiding the consumption of fatty, processed or sugary foods.

How to maintain my budget with the DASH Diet?

There is a myth that a good diet is expensive and it is not so, the DASH diet is an affordable diet for everyone and with a fully controllable budget. In addition to investing in a good diet, is investing in health, eliminating the costs of medical consultations, medicines and even preventable surgical interventions.

Besides, you should know that this diet is not a fad, it is a diet supported by specialists and institutions such as the American Heart Association, American Cancer Society, among others.

The foods that you should consume for this diet are basic and healthy products such as: fruits, vegetables, nuts, whole grains, fat-free or low-fat dairy products, fish, among others. Keep in mind that by having this cookbook in your hands you can easily plan your shopping and make a budget for each purchase. This way you will take care of your finances and your health.

What are the benefits of the DASH Diet?

The DASH diet has multiple benefits, the most popular is that it prevents hypertension, but it is also a great aid in preventing heart disease, heart failure and stroke, osteoporosis, is an ally in menopause, reduces and improves cholesterol levels, prevents or controls type II diabetes, reduces the likelihood of kidney stones and if that were not enough, it is also excellent for weight loss, so you will be healthier and fitter. As you will see the DASH diet is an excellent deal, better health, more fit, savings on medical visits and treatments and a budget under control.

Chapter 2 -   Breakfast Recipes

1) *Complete Cheesy Breakfast Egg*

Preparation Time: 15 minutes

Cooking Time: 41 minutes

Servings: 4-6

Nutrition: Calories: 337 Carbs: 17g Fat: 25g Protein: 12g

Ingredients:

- 6 large eggs
- 3 tbsp extra-virgin olive oil
- 1 large onion, halved and thinly sliced
- 1 large red bell pepper, seeded and thinly sliced
- 3 garlic cloves, thinly sliced
- 1 tsp ground cumin
- 1 tsp sweet paprika
- 1/8 tsp cayenne, or to taste
- 1 (28-ounce) can whole plum tomatoes with juices, coarsely chopped
- ¼ tsp black pepper, more as needed
- 5 oz feta cheese, crumbled, about 1 1/4 cups
- To Serve:
- Chopped cilantro
- Hot sauce

Directions:

❖ Preheat oven to 375 degrees F. In a large skillet over medium-low heat, add the oil. Once heated, add the onion and bell pepper, cook gently until very soft, about 20 minutes.

❖ Add in the garlic and cook until tender, 1 to 2 minutes, then stir in cumin, paprika and cayenne, and cook 1 minute.

❖ Pour in tomatoes, season with 1/4 tsp pepper, simmer until tomatoes have thickened, about 10 minutes. Then stir in crumbled feta.

❖ Gently crack eggs into skillet over tomatoes, season with pepper. Transfer skillet to oven. Bake until eggs have just set, 7 to 10 minutes. Serve.

2) *Vegetables Spicy Frittata*

Preparation Time: 15 minutes

Cooking Time: 15 minutes

Servings: 2

Nutrition: Calories: 271, Fats: 5.2g, Carbs: 44.7g, Proteins: 18.2g,

Ingredients:

- 8 ounces fresh asparagus, trimmed and cut into 1-inch pieces
- ¼ of red bell pepper, seeded
- ¼ of green bell pepper, seeded
- 1 tablespoon fresh chives, chopped
- ¾ cup water
- ½ cup superfine chickpea flour
- 1 tablespoon chia seeds
- 2 tablespoons nutritional yeast
- ½ teaspoon baking powder
- 1 teaspoon dried basil, crushed
- ¼ teaspoon ground turmeric
- ¼ teaspoon red pepper flakes, crushed
- Ground black pepper, as required
- 1 small tomato, chopped

Directions:

❖ In a pan of the lightly salted boiling water, add the asparagus and Cooking Time: for about 5-7 minutes or until crisp tender.

❖ Drain the asparagus well and set aside.

❖ Meanwhile, in a bowl, add the bell peppers, chives and water and mix.

❖ In another bowl, add the remaining ingredients except tomato and mix well.

❖ Add the water mixture into the bowl of flour mixture and mix until well combined.

❖ Set aside for at least 10 minutes.

❖ Lightly, grease a large nonstick skillet and heat over medium heat

3) *Yellow Greek Yogurt with Peanut Cream*

Preparation Time: 15 minutes

Cooking Time: 0 minutes

Servings: 4

Nutrition: Calories: 370 Carbs: 47g Fat: 10g Protein: 22g

Ingredients:

- 3 cups vanilla Greek yogurt
- 2 medium bananas sliced
- 1/4 cup creamy natural peanut butter
- 1/4 cup flaxseed meal
- 1 tsp nutmeg

Directions:

❖ Divide yogurt between four jars with lids. Top with banana slices.

❖ In a bowl, melt the peanut butter in a microwave safe bowl for 30-40 seconds and drizzle one tbsp on each bowl on top of the bananas. Store in the fridge for up to 3 days.

❖ When ready to serve, sprinkle with flaxseed meal and ground nutmeg. Enjoy!

4) *Superfood Bars with Apple Sauce*

Preparation Time: 15 minutes

Cooking Time: 40 minutes

Servings: 12

Nutrition: Calories: 230 Fat: 10g Carbs: 31g Protein: 7g

Ingredients:

- 2 eggs
- 1 apple peeled and chopped into ½ inch chunks
- 1 cup unsweetened apple sauce
- 1 ½ cups cooked & cooled quinoa
- 1 ½ cups rolled oats
- 1/4 cup peanut butter
- 1 tsp vanilla
- 1/2 tsp cinnamon
- 1/4 cup coconut oil
- ½ tsp baking powder

Directions:

❖ Heat oven to 350 degrees F. Spray an 8x8 inch baking dish with oil, set aside. In a large bowl, stir together the apple sauce, cinnamon, coconut oil, peanut butter, vanilla and eggs.

❖ Add in the cooked quinoa, rolled oats and baking powder, mix until completely incorporated. Fold in the apple chunks.

❖ Spread the mixture into the prepared baking dish, spreading it to each corner. Bake for 40 minutes, or until a toothpick comes out clean. Allow to cool before slicing.

5) *Tofu and Broccoli Quiche*

Preparation Time: 15 minutes

Cooking Time: 15 minutes

Servings: 2

Nutrition: Calories: 212, Fats: 10.4g, Carbs: 19.6g, Proteins: 14.4g,

Ingredients:

- 1 cup water
- 1/3 cup bulgur wheat
- ¾ tablespoon light sesame oil
- 1½ cups fresh cremini mushrooms, sliced
- 2 cups fresh broccoli, chopped
- 1 yellow onion, chopped
- 16 ounces firm tofu, pressed and cubed
- ¾ tablespoon white miso
- 1¼ tablespoons tahini
- 1 tablespoon soy sauce

Directions:

- ❖ Preheat the oven to 350 degrees F. Grease a pie dish.
- ❖ In a pan, add the water over medium heat bring to a boil.
- ❖ Stir in the bulgur and again bring to a boil.
- ❖ Reduce the heat to low and simmer, covered for about 12-15 minutes or until all the liquid is absorbed.
- ❖ Remove from the heat and let it cool slightly.
- ❖ Now, place the cooked bulgur into the pie dish evenly and with your fingers, press into the bottom.
- ❖ Bake for about 12 minutes.
- ❖ Remove from the oven and let it cool slightly.
- ❖ Meanwhile, in a skillet, heat oil over medium heat.
- ❖ Add the mushrooms, broccoli and onion and Cooking Time: for about 10 minutes, stirring occasionally.
- ❖ Remove from the heat and transfer into a large bowl to cool slightly.
- ❖ Meanwhile, in a food processor, add the remaining ingredients and pulse until smooth.
- ❖ Transfer the tofu mixture into the bowl with veggie mixture and mix until well combined.
- ❖ Place the veggie mixture over the baked crust evenly.
- ❖ Bake for about 30 minutes or until top becomes golden brown.
- ❖ Remove from the oven and set aside for at least 10 minutes.
- ❖ With a sharp knife, cut into 4 equal sized slices and serve.
- ❖ Meal Preparation time: Tip:
- ❖ In a reseal able plastic bag, place the cooled quiche slices and seal the bag.
- ❖ Refrigerate for about 2-4 days.
- ❖ Reheat in the microwave on High for about 1 minute before serving.

6) *Red and Full Breakfast Tortillas*

Preparation Time: 15 minutes

Cooking Time: 15 minutes

Servings: 5

Nutrition: Calories: 213 Fat: 11g Carbs: 15g Protein: 15g

Ingredients:

- 8 eggs (optional)
- 2 tsp olive oil
- 1 red bell pepper
- 1/2 red onion
- 1/4 cup milk
- 4 handfuls of spinach leaves
- 1 1/2 cup mozzarella cheese
- 5 sun-dried tomato tortillas
- 1/2 cup feta
- 1/4 tsp pepper
- Spray oil

Direction:

- ❖ In a large non-stick pan over medium heat, add the olive oil. Once heated, add the bell pepper and onion, cook for 4-5 minutes until soft. In the meantime, whisk together the eggs, milk and pepper in a bowl. Add in the egg/milk mixture into the pan with peppers and onions, stirring frequently, until eggs are almost cooked through.
- ❖ Add in the spinach and feta, fold into the eggs, stirring until spinach is wilted and eggs are cooked through. Remove the eggs from heat and plate.
- ❖ Spray a separate large non-stick pan with spray oil, and place over medium heat. Add the tortilla, on one half of the tortilla, spread about ½ cup of the egg mixture.
- ❖ Top the eggs with around 1/3 cup of shredded mozzarella cheese. Fold the second half of the tortilla over, then cook for 2 minutes, or until golden brown.
- ❖ Flip and cook for another minute until golden brown. Allow the quesadilla to cool completely, divide among the container, store for 2 days or wrap in plastic wrap and foil, and freeze for up to 2 months

7) _Deli Maple Bread_

Preparation Time: 15 minutes

Cooking Time: 40 minutes

Servings: 16

Nutrition: Calories: 118, Fats: 0.3g, Carbs: 24.7g, Proteins: 3.5g,

Ingredients:

- 2 teaspoons maple syrup
- 2 cups warm water
- 4 cups whole-wheat flour
- 1 tablespoon instant yeast

Directions:

- ❖ In a cup, dissolve the maple syrup in warm water.
- ❖ In a large bowl, add the flour, yeast and mix well.
- ❖ Add the maple syrup mixture and mix until a sticky dough forms.
- ❖ Transfer the dough into a greased 9×5-inch loaf pan.
- ❖ Cover the loaf pan and set aside for about 20 minutes.
- ❖ Preheat the oven to 390 degrees F.
- ❖ Uncover the loaf pan and bake for about 40 minutes or until a toothpick inserted in the center comes out clean.
- ❖ Remove the pan from oven and place onto a wire rack to cool for about 20 minutes.
- ❖ Carefully, remove the bread from the loaf pan and place onto the wire rack to cool completely before slicing.
- ❖ With a sharp knife, cut the bread loaf into desired sized slices and serve.
- ❖ Meal Preparation time: Tip:
- ❖ In a resealable plastic bag, place the bread and seal the bag after squeezing out the excess air.
- ❖ Keep the bread away from direct sunlight and preserve in a cool and dry place for about 1-2 days.

8) _Olive Muffins Quinoa with Feta and Cherry_

Preparation Time: 15 minutes

Cooking Time: 30 minutes

Servings: 12

Nutrition: Calories: 113 Carbs: 5g Fat: 7g Protein: 6g

Ingredients:

- 8 eggs
- 1 cup cooked quinoa
- 1 cup crumbled feta cheese
- 2 cups baby spinach finely chopped
- 1/2 cup finely chopped onion
- 1 cup chopped or sliced tomatoes, cherry or grape tomatoes
- 1/2 cup chopped and pitted Kalamata olives
- 1 tbsp chopped fresh oregano
- 2 tsp high oleic sunflower oil plus optional extra for greasing muffin tins

Direction:

- ❖ Pre-heat oven to 350 degrees F. Prepare 12 silicone muffin holders on a baking sheet, or grease a 12-cup muffin tin with oil, set aside.
- ❖ In a skillet over medium heat, add the vegetable oil and onions, sauté for 2 minutes. Add tomatoes, sauté for another minute, then add spinach and sauté until wilted, about 1 minute.
- ❖ Remove from heat and stir in olives and oregano, set aside. Place the eggs in a blender or mixing bowl and blend or mix until well combined.
- ❖ Pour the eggs in to a mixing bowl (if you used a blender) then add quinoa, feta cheese, veggie mixture and stir until well combined.
- ❖ Pour mixture in to silicone cups or greased muffin tins, dividing equally, and bake for 30 minutes, or until eggs have set and muffins are a light golden brown. Allow to cool completely.

9) _Orange Coco Shake_

Preparation Time: 5 minutes

Cooking Time: 0 minute

Servings: 1

Nutrition: Calories: 335 Fat: 5 g Carbs: 75 g Protein: 4 g

Ingredients:

- 1 tablespoon coconut flakes
- 1 1/2 cups frozen banana slices
- 8 strawberries, sliced
- 1/2 cup coconut milk, unsweetened
- 1/4 cup strawberries for topping

Directions:

- ❖ Place all the ingredients in the order in a food processor or blender, except for topping and then pulse for 2 to 3 minutes at high speed until smooth.
- ❖ Pour the smoothie into a glass and then serve.

10) Sweety Avena Fruit Muffins with Walnuts

Preparation Time: 15 minutes

Cooking Time: 15 minutes

Servings: 6

Nutrition: Calories: 351, Fats: 14.4g, Carbs: 51.8g, Proteins: 8.2g,

Ingredients:

- ½ cup hot water
- ¼ cup ground flaxseeds
- 1 banana, peeled and sliced
- 1 apple, peeled, cored and chopped roughly
- 2 cups rolled oats
- ½ cup walnuts, chopped
- ½ cup raisins
- ¼ teaspoon baking soda
- 2 tablespoons ground cinnamon
- ½ cup almond milk
- ¼ cup maple syrup

Directions:

- ❖ Preheat the oven to 350 degrees F. Line a 12 cups muffin tin with paper liners.
- ❖ In a bowl, add water and flaxseed and beat until well combined. Set aside for about 5 minutes.
- ❖ In a blender, add the flaxseed mixture and remaining all ingredients except blueberries and pulse till smooth and creamy.
- ❖ Transfer the mixture into prepared muffin cups evenly.
- ❖ Bake for about 20 minutes or until a toothpick inserted in the center comes out clean.
- ❖ Remove the muffin tin from oven and place onto a wire rack to cool for about 10 minutes.
- ❖ Carefully invert the muffins onto the wire rack to cool completely before serving.
- ❖ Meal Preparation time: Tip:
- ❖ Carefully invert the muffins onto a wire rack to cool completely.
- ❖ Line 1-2 airtight containers with paper towels.
- ❖ Arrange muffins over paper towel in a single layer.
- ❖ Cover the muffins with another paper towel.
- ❖ Refrigerate for about 2-3 days.
- ❖ Reheat in the microwave on High for about 2 minutes before serving.

11) Cheesy Muffins with Mushroom and Herbs

Preparation Time: 20 minutes

Cooking Time: 20 minutes

Servings: 6

Nutrition: Calories: 74, Fats: 3.5g, Carbs: 5.3g, Proteins: 6.2g,

Ingredients:

- 1 teaspoon olive oil
- 1½ cups fresh mushrooms, chopped
- 1 scallion, chopped
- 1 teaspoon garlic, minced
- 1 teaspoon fresh rosemary, minced
- Ground black pepper, as required
- 1 (12.3-ouncepackage lite firm silken tofu, drained
- ¼ cup unsweetened almond milk
- 2 tablespoons nutritional yeast
- 1 tablespoon arrowroot starch
- 1 teaspoon coconut oil, softened
- ¼ teaspoon ground turmeric

Directions:

- ❖ Preheat the oven to 375 degrees F. Grease a 12 cups of a muffin pan.
- ❖ In a nonstick skillet, heat the oil over medium heat and sauté the scallion and garlic for about 1 minute.
- ❖ Add the mushrooms and sauté for about 5-7 minutes.
- ❖ Stir in the rosemary and black pepper and remove from the heat.
- ❖ Set aside to cool slightly.
- ❖ In a food processor, add the tofu and remaining ingredients and pulse until smooth.
- ❖ Transfer the tofu mixture into a large bowl.
- ❖ Fold in the mushroom mixture.
- ❖ Place the mixture into prepared muffin cups evenly.
- ❖ Bake for about 20-22 minutes or until a toothpick inserted in the center comes out clean.
- ❖ Remove the muffin pan from the oven and place onto a wire rack to cool for about 10 minutes.
- ❖ Carefully, invert the muffins onto wire rack and serve warm.
- ❖ Meal Preparation time: Tip:
- ❖ Carefully invert the muffins onto a wire rack to cool completely.
- ❖ Line 1-2 airtight containers with paper towels.
- ❖ Arrange muffins over paper towel in a single layer.
- ❖ Cover the muffins with another paper towel.
- ❖ Refrigerate for about 2-3 days.

12) *Green Banana Shake with Vanilla*

Preparation Time: 5 minutes

Cooking Time: 0 minute

Servings: 1

Nutrition: Calories: 298 Fat: 11 g Carbs: 32 g Protein: 24 g

Ingredients:

- 1 teaspoon flax seeds
- 1 frozen banana
- 1 cup baby spinach
- 1/2 teaspoon ground cinnamon
- 1/4 teaspoon vanilla extract, unsweetened
- 2 tablespoons peanut butter, unsweetened
- 1/4 cup ice
- 1 cup coconut milk, unsweetened

Directions:

- Place all the ingredients in the order in a food processor or blender and then pulse for 2 to 3 minutes at high speed until smooth.
- Pour the smoothie into a glass and then serve.

13) *Healthy Breakfast Frittata*

Preparation Time: 8 minutes

Cooking Time: 6 minutes

Servings: 4

Nutrition: Calories: 178 Protein: 16 g Fat: 12 g Carbs: 2.2 g

Ingredients:

- 2 teaspoons of olive oil
- 3/4 cup of baby spinach, packed
- 2 green onions
- 4 egg whites, large
- 6 large eggs
- 1/3 cup of crumbled feta cheese, (1.3 ounces) along with sun-dried tomatoes and basil
- 2 teaspoons of salt-free Greek seasoning

Directions:

- Take a boiler and preheat it. Take a ten-inch ovenproof skillet and pour the oil into it and keep the skillet on a medium flame.
- While the oil gets heated, chop the spinach roughly and the onions. Put the eggs, egg whites, Greek seasoning, cheese, as well as salt in a large mixing bowl and mix it thoroughly using a whisker.
- Add the chopped spinach and onions into the mixing bowl and stir it well.
- Pour the mixture into the pan and cook it for 2 minutes or more until the edges of the mixture set well.
- Lift the edges of the mixture gently and tilt the pan so that the uncooked portion can get underneath it. Cook for another two minutes so that the whole mixture gets cooked properly.
- Broil for two to three minutes till the center gets set. Your Frittata is now ready. Serve it hot by cutting it into four wedges.

14) *Good Mexican Style Tortilla*

Preparation Time: 10 minutes

Cooking Time:

Servings: 6

Nutrition: Calories: 157 Carbs: 4.2g Fat: 13.8g Protein: 5.0g

Ingredients:

- ¼ cup ground flaxseed
- ¼ cup hot water
- 1 cup almond flour
- ¼ tsp. baking powder

Directions:

- Mix ground flaxseed with hot water until you get a gel-like substance.
- In a separate bowl, mix almond flour and baking powder.
- Add ground flaxseed mixture to almond flour mixture.
- Mix thoroughly.
- Add hot water as needed in order to achieve a perfect dough-like consistency.
- Knead dough, then separate dough into about 6 balls.
- Flatten each ball as thinly as possible.
- Grease a pan.
- Place each tortilla on greased pan and bake each tortilla until brown on both sides.
- Remove pan from oven.
- Let cool completely before using as they are easier to mold and fold once cool.
- This bread-based recipe comes in handy if you're craving a good old tofu wrap or even a vegan-styled quesadilla!

15) Coco Peach Oats Shake

Preparation Time: 5 minutes

Cooking Time: 0 minute

Servings: 1

Nutrition: Calories: 270 Fat: 4 g Carbs: 28 g Protein: 25 g

Ingredients:

- 1 tablespoon chia seeds
- ¼ cup rolled oats
- 2 peaches, pitted, sliced
- ¾ teaspoon ground cinnamon
- 1 Medjool date, pitted
- ½ teaspoon vanilla extract, unsweetened
- 2 tablespoons lemon juice
- ½ cup of water
- 1 tablespoon coconut butter
- 1 cup coconut milk, unsweetened

Directions:

- ❖ Place all the ingredients in the order in a food processor or blender and then pulse for 2 to 3 minutes at high speed until smooth.
- ❖ Pour the smoothie into a glass and then serve.

16) Spicy Queso Pizza with Avocado Flavour

Preparation Time: 20 minutes

Cooking Time: 20 minutes

Servings: 2

Nutrition: Calories: 416 Protein: 15 g Fat: 10 g Carbs: 37 g

Ingredients:

- 1 and 1/4 cups of chickpea or garbanzo bean flour
- 1 and 1/4 cups of cold water
- 1/4 teaspoon of pepper
- 2 teaspoons of avocado or olive oil + 1 teaspoon extra for heating the pan
- 1 teaspoon of minced Garlic which will be around two cloves
- 1 teaspoon of Onion powder/other herb seasoning powder
- 10 to twelve-inch cast iron pan
- 1 sliced tomato
- 1/2 avocado
- 2 ounces of thinly sliced Gouda
- 1/4-1/3 cup of Tomato sauce
- 2 or 3 teaspoons of chopped green scallion/onion
- Sprouted greens for green
- Extra pepper for sprinkling on top of the pizza
- Red pepper flakes

Directions:

- ❖ Mix the flour with two teaspoons of olive oil, herbs, water, and whisk it until a smooth mixture form. Keep it at room temperature for around 15-20 minutes to let the batter settle.
- ❖ In the meantime, preheat the oven and place the pan inside the oven and let it get heated for around 10 minutes. When the pan gets preheated, chop up the vegetables into fine slices.
- ❖ Remove the pan after ten minutes using oven mitts. Put one teaspoon of oil and swirl it all around to coat the pan.
- ❖ Pour the batter into the pan and tilt the pan so that the batter spreads evenly throughout the pan. Turn down the over to 425f and place back the pan for 5-8 minutes.
- ❖ Remove the pan from the oven and add the sliced avocado, tomato and on top of that, add the gouda slices and the onion slices.
- ❖ Put the pizza back into the oven and wait till the cheese get melted or the sides of the bread gets crusty and brown.
- ❖ Remove the pizza from the pan and add the microgreens on top, along with the toppings.

17) Baked Seed Mix Loaf

Preparation Time: 15 minutes

Cooking Time:

Servings: 15

Nutrition: Calories: 172 Carbs: 8.1g Fat: 13.2g Protein: 6.1g

Ingredients:

- 2 cups almond flour
- 2 tbsp. coconut flour
- ⅓ cup coconut oil
- ½ cup whole almonds
- 3 tbsp. sesame seeds
- ½ cup pumpkin seeds
- ¼ cup whole flax seeds
- 3 flax eggs
- 1 ½ tsp. baking soda
- ¾ cup almond milk
- 3 drops stevia sweetener
- 1 tbsp. apple cider vinegar Total number of ingredients: 13

Directions:

- ❖ Preheat oven to 350 °F.
- ❖ Blend almonds in a blender until fine.
- ❖ Add flax seeds, sesame seeds, and pumpkin seeds and blend.
- ❖ Add almond flour, coconut flour, and baking soda and blend.
- ❖ In a separate bowl, add flax eggs, coconut oil, almond milk, vinegar, and sweetener. Stir well.
- ❖ Add almond mixture to flax egg mixture and let sit for a few minutes.
- ❖ Grease a loaf pan.
- ❖ Pour batter in pan.
- ❖ Sprinkle left over seeds atop batter (pumpkin, flax, and sesame seeds).
- ❖ Bake for about 45 minutes, or until a knife comes clean out of the middle.
- ❖ Remove from oven, and let cool completely before slicing.

18) Almond Corn Bread with Coconut Oil

Preparation Time: 10 minutes

Cooking Time:

Servings: 18

Nutrition: Calories 138 Carbs: 7.2g Fat: 10.7g Protein: 3.5g

Ingredients:
- 2 cups almond flour
- 6 drops stevia sweetener
- 2 flax eggs
- 3 ½ tsp. baking powder
- ½ cup vanilla flavored almond milk
- ⅓ cup coconut oil
- 15 oz. can baby corn, finely chopped Total number of ingredients: 8

Directions:
- ❖ Preheat oven to 350 °F.
- ❖ In a bowl, mix almond flour, and baking powder.
- ❖ Add stevia, chopped corn, flax eggs, almond milk, and coconut oil.
- ❖ Mix well, ensuring no clumps.
- ❖ Lightly grease a pan.
- ❖ Pour batter in pan.
- ❖ Place pan in oven and let bake 50-60 minutes or until knife comes cleanly out of the middle.

19) Delicious Breakfast Seed Crackers

Preparation Time: 5 minutes

Cooking Time:

Servings: 25 crackers

Nutrition: Calories: 53 Carbs: 3.5g Fat: 3.6g Protein: 1.6g

Ingredients:
- 1 cup flaxseed, ground
- 1 cup pumpkin seeds
- ½ cup sesame seeds
- 1 cup hot water

Directions:
- ❖ Preheat oven to 300 °F.
- ❖ Place all ingredients in a bowl and mix.
- ❖ Let sit for five minutes (the flaxseed will form a gel with the water).
- ❖ Spread mixture on a parchment paper-lined pan.
- ❖ Using a knife, cut dough evenly into about 25 crackers.
- ❖ Place in oven and bake until firm.
- ❖ Turn oven off, leaving crackers in oven for about 1 hour so that crackers dry out.

20) Berries Mix Mug Bread

Preparation Time: 3 minutes

Cooking Time:

Servings: 4 slices

Nutrition: Calories: 165 Carbs: 25.5g Fat: 6.2g Protein: 4.1g

Ingredients:
- ⅓ cup almond flour (or any other nut flour of your preference
- 1 flax egg
- ¼ tsp. baking soda
- 2 tbsp. of your desired dried fruit (For this recipe, raspberries and strawberries were chosen

Directions:
- ❖ To a bowl, add almond flour, baking soda and dried fruits. Mix thoroughly.
- ❖ Add flax egg and stir until evenly distributed. Also make sure dried fruits are evenly distributed in the batter.
- ❖ Lightly grease a mug that is big enough to hold batter.
- ❖ Pour batter into mug and microwave for about 2 minutes.
- ❖ Remove mug from oven, and slice mini loaf into about 4 pieces.

Chapter 3 -   Rice, Grain and Pasta Recipes

21) *Cheesy Fettuccini with Tomatoes and Chicken*

Preparation Time: 5 minutes

Cooking Time: 30 minutes

Servings: 6

Nutrition: Calories: 390 Protein: 19 g Fat: 11 g Carbs: 56 g

Ingredients:

- 2-tbsp extra-virgin olive oil
- 1½-lb chicken breasts, boneless, skinless, and split in half
- ¼-tsp freshly ground black pepper
- 2-cups water
- 2-14.5-oz. cans diced tomatoes with basil, garlic, and oregano
- 1-lb whole-wheat fettuccini pasta
- 4-oz. reduced-fat feta cheese (divided)
- Fresh basil leaves, finely chopped (optional)

Directions:

- ❖ Heat the olive oil for 1 minute in your Dutch oven placed over high heat for 1 minute. Add the chicken, and sprinkle over with freshly ground black pepper.
- ❖ Cook the chicken for 8 minutes, flipping once. Cook further for 5 minutes until the chicken cooks through.
- ❖ Pour in the water, and add the tomatoes. Stir in the fettuccini pasta, cook for 5 minutes, uncovered. Cover the dish, and cook further for 10 minutes.
- ❖ Uncover the dish, and stir the pasta. Add 3-oz. of the feta cheese, and stir again. Cook further for 5 minutes, uncovered. To serve, sprinkle over with the chopped basil and the remaining feta cheese.

22) *Chickpeas Hummus Pasta*

Preparation Time: 30 minutes

Cooking Time:

Servings: 2

Nutrition: Carbs: 61.8g Protein: 18.9g Fats: 18.9g Calories: 488

Ingredients:

- 'Pasta: 1 cup
- Olive oil: 1 tbsp
- Chickpeas: 1 cup can
- Garlic: 2 cloves minced
- Garlic: 1 tbsp minced
- Red onion: 1 small diced
- Cumin: 1 tsp
- Pepper: ½ tsp
- Hummus: ½ cup

Directions:

- ❖ Cooking Time: pasta as per packet instructions
- ❖ Take a large saucepan and add olive oil and heat on medium flame
- ❖ Include onion, ginger, and garlic to the pan and Cooking Time: for 2-4 minutes
- ❖ Now add chickpeas, cumin, and pepper
- ❖ Stir the spoon and add pasta
- ❖ Lower the heat and cover and Cooking Time: for 2 minutes and mix in hummus and serve

23) *Delicious Fruity Pasta*

Preparation Time: 5 minutes

Cooking Time: 10 minutes

Servings: 6

Nutrition: Calories: 329 Protein: 12 g Fat: 13 g Carbs: 43 g

Ingredients:

- 4-quarts water
- 10-oz. gluten-free and whole-grain pasta
- 5-cloves garlic, minced
- 1-cup hummus
- Pepper
- 1/3-cup water
- ½-cup walnuts
- ½-cup olives
- 2-tbsp dried cranberries

Directions:

- ❖ Bring the water to a boil for cooking the pasta.
- ❖ In the meantime, prepare for the hummus sauce. Combine the garlic, hummus, and pepper with water in a mixing bowl. Add the walnuts, olive, and dried cranberries. Set aside.
- ❖ Add the pasta in the boiling water. Cook the pasta following the manufacturer's specifications until attaining an al dente texture. Drain the pasta. Transfer the pasta to a large serving bowl and combine with the sauce.

24) *Black Beans and Zucchini Pasta with Cilantro*

Preparation Time: 30 minutes

Cooking Time:

Servings: 2

Nutrition: Carbs: 28.15g Protein: 12.35g Fats: 8.5g Calories: 287

Ingredients:

- Pasta: 1 cup (after cooked
- Olive oil: 1 tbsp
- Vegetable broth: ½ cup
- Black beans: 1 cup
- Garlic: 2 cloves minced
- Zucchini: 1 cup diced
- Red onion: 1 small diced
- Chili powder: 1 tsp
- Cumin: 1 tsp
- Black pepper: ½ tsp
- Fresh cilantro: 2 tbsp

Directions:

- ❖ Take a large saucepan and add olive oil and heat on medium flame
- ❖ Include onion and garlic to the pan and Cooking Time: for a minute
- ❖ Now add zucchini, black beans, cumin, chili powder, and broth
- ❖ Stir the spoon and let them boil
- ❖ Lower the heat and cover and Cooking Time: for 10 minutes
- ❖ In the meanwhile, Cooking Time: pasta as per packet instructions
- ❖ When done, add to the beans
- ❖ Sprinkle pepper and cilantro on top and serve

25) *Italian Pappardelle with Jumbo Shrimp*

Preparation Time: 10 minutes

Cooking Time: 20 minutes

Servings: 4

Nutrition: Calories: 474 Protein: 37 g Fat: 15 g Carbs: 46 g

Ingredients:

- 3-quarts water
- 1-lb. jumbo shrimp, peeled and deveined
- ¼-tsp black pepper, freshly grated
- 3-tbsp olive oil (divided)
- 2-cups zucchini, cut diagonally to ⅛-inch thick slices
- 1-cup grape tomatoes halved
- 1/8-tsp red pepper flakes
- 2-cloves garlic, minced
- 1 tsp zest of 1-pc lemon
- 2-tbsp lemon juice
- 1-tbsp Italian parsley, chopped
- 8-oz. fresh pappardelle pasta

Directions:

- ❖ Bring the water to a boil for cooking the pasta. In the meantime, prepare for the shrimp. Combine the shrimp with pepper. Set aside.
- ❖ Heat a tablespoon of oil in a large sauté pan placed over medium heat. Add the zucchini slices and sauté for 4 minutes until they are tender.
- ❖ Add the grape tomatoes and sauté for 2 minutes until they just start to soften. Stir in the salt to combine with the vegetables. Transfer the cooked vegetables to a medium-sized bowl. Set aside.
- ❖ In the same sauté pan, pour in the remaining oil. Switch the heat to medium-low. Add the red pepper flakes and garlic. Cook for 2 minutes, stirring frequently so that the garlic will not burn.
- ❖ Add the seasoned shrimp, and keep the heat on medium-low. Cook the shrimp for 3 minutes on each side until they turn pinkish.
- ❖ Stir in the zest of lemon and the lemon juice. Add the cooked vegetables back to the pan. Stir to combine with the shrimp. Set aside.
- ❖ Add the pasta in the boiling water. Cook the pasta following the manufacturer's specifications until attaining an al dente texture. Drain the pasta.
- ❖ Transfer the cooked pasta in a large serving bowl and combine with the lemony-garlic shrimp and vegetables.

26) *Spaghetti with Salsa "Arrabbiata"*

Preparation Time: 15 minutes

Cooking Time:

Servings: 2

Nutrition: Carbs: 21.8g Protein: 8.45g Fats: 15.95g Calories: 379

Ingredients:

- Spaghetti: 1 cup (after cooking
- Cherry tomatoes: 4 halved
- Spring onions: 3 chopped
- Garlic: 3 cloves minced
- Vinegar: 3 tbsp
- Olive oil: 2 tbsp
- Tabasco: 5 dashes
- Pepper: as per your taste
- Basil: 2 tbsp torn

Directions:

- ❖ Take a bowl and add in cherry tomatoes, minced garlic, olive oil, vinegar, Tabasco, spring onion, and a lot of pepper
- ❖ Cooking Time: spaghetti as per packet instructions
- ❖ Drain the pasta but keep 2 tablespoons of water and add to the sauce
- ❖ Blend the sauce by removing tomatoes
- ❖ Add pasta to the sauce and mix in tomatoes
- ❖ Top with basil and serve

27) *Creamy Pasta and Broccoli*

Preparation Time: 30 minutes

Cooking Time:

Servings: 2

Nutrition: Carbs: 26.2g Protein: 6.7g Fats: 9.65g Calories: 204

Ingredients:

- Pasta: 1 cup (after cooking
- Broccoli florets: 1 cup
- Olive oil: 1 tbsp
- Cashew cream: ½ cup
- Green onion: 1 chopped
- Pepper: as per your taste

Directions:

- ❖ Cooking Time: pasta as per packet instructions
- ❖ Preheat the oven to 400F
- ❖ In a bowl, add broccoli and season with pepper and brush with oil
- ❖ Add them to the baking sheet and roast for 20 minutes
- ❖ In a serving tray, spread pasta and top with roasted broccoli
- ❖ Spread cashew cream on top
- ❖ Sprinkle green onions on top and serve

28) Sicilian Linguine with Mushroom Mix

Preparation Time: 5 minutes

Cooking Time: 30 minutes

Servings: 8

Nutrition: Calories: 331 Protein: 13 g Fat: 12 g Carbs: 45 g

Ingredients:

- 5-quarts water
- 3-tbsp olive oil
- 26-oz. assorted wild mushrooms (Crimini, Shiitake, Portobello, etc.), sliced
- 4-cloves garlic, minced
- 1-bulb red onion, diced
- 2-tbsp sherry cooking wine
- 2½-tsp fresh thyme, diced
- 1-lb. linguine pasta
- ¾-cup reserved liquid from cooked pasta
- 6-oz. goat cheese
- ¼-cup hazelnuts, chopped

Directions:

- ❖ Bring the water to a boil for cooking the pasta. In the meantime, heat the olive oil in a large skillet placed over medium-high heat. Add the mushrooms and sauté for 10 minutes until they brown.
- ❖ Add the garlic and onions. Sauté for 4 minutes until the onions are translucent. Pour in the wine, and cook down until the liquid evaporates. Sprinkle with thyme, and set aside.
- ❖ Add the pasta in the boiling water. Cook the pasta following the manufacturer's specifications until attaining an al dente texture. Before draining the pasta completely, reserve ¾-cup of the pasta liquid.
- ❖ Transfer the cooked pasta in a large serving bowl and combine with the mushroom mixture, pasta liquid, and goat cheese.
- ❖ Toss gently to combine fully until the goat cheese melts completely. To serve, top the pasta with chopped hazelnuts.

29) Tomato Pasta with Parmesan Cheese

Preparation Time: 5 minutes

Cooking Time: 20 minutes

Servings: 4

Nutrition: Calories: 265 Protein: 12 g Fat: 15 g Carbs: 17 g

Ingredients:

- 8 ounces whole-grain linguine
- 1 tablespoon extra-virgin olive oil
- 2 garlic cloves, minced
- 1/4 cup chopped yellow onion
- 1 teaspoon chopped fresh oregano
- 1/4 teaspoon freshly ground black pepper
- 1 teaspoon tomato paste
- 8 ounces cherry tomatoes, halved
- 1/2 cup grated Parmesan cheese
- 1 tablespoon chopped fresh parsley

Directions:

- ❖ Bring a large saucepan of water to a boil over high heat and cook the linguine according to the package instructions until al dente (still slightly firm). Drain, reserving 1/2 cup of the pasta water. Do not rinse the pasta.
- ❖ In a large, heavy skillet, heat the olive oil over medium-high heat. Sauté the garlic, onion, and oregano until the onion is just translucent, about 5 minutes.
- ❖ Add the salt, pepper, tomato paste, and 1/4 cup of the reserved pasta water. Stir well and allow it to cook for 1 minute.
- ❖ Stir in the tomatoes and cooked pasta, tossing everything well to coat. Add more pasta water if needed.

30) Veggie Mix Pasta with Mustard Dressing

Preparation Time: 30 minutes

Cooking Time:

Servings: 4

Nutrition: Carbs: 41.5g Protein: 10.7g Fats: 8.1g Calories: 399

Ingredients:

- Macaroni pasta: 4 cups
- Carrots: 1 cup sliced
- Broccoli: 1 cup sliced
- Cauliflower: 1 cup sliced
- Olive oil: 1 tbsp
- Pepper: as per your taste
- For the Dressing:
- Lemon: 2 zest and juice
- Mustard: 1 tbsp
- Vinegar: 2 tsp
- Garlic: 1 clove crushed
- Extra-virgin olive oil: 2 tbsp

Directions:

- ❖ Cooking Time: pasta as per packet instructions
- ❖ Add all the vegetables to the baking tray, sprinkle pepper, brush with olive oil and bake for 20 minutes
- ❖ Prepare the dressing by adding all the ingredients except oil and combine it slowly at the end whisking to gain the correct consistency
- ❖ Add pasta to the tray, and spread vegetables to the tray and pour dressing from the top and serve

31) Pasta with "Cacciatora" Sauce

Preparation Time: 10 minutes

Cooking Time: 17 minutes

Servings: 4

Nutrition: Calories 615 Fat 15.4 g Carbs 71 g Protein 48 g

Ingredients:

- 3 chicken breasts, skinless, boneless, cut into pieces
- 9 oz whole-grain pasta
- 1/2 cup olives, sliced
- 1/2 cup sun-dried tomatoes
- 1 tbsp roasted red peppers, chopped
- 14 oz can tomato, diced
- 2 cups marinara sauce
- 1 cup chicken broth
- Pepper

Directions:

- ❖ Add all ingredients except whole-grain pasta into the instant pot and stir well. Seal pot with lid and cook on high for 12 minutes.
- ❖ Once done, allow to release pressure naturally. Remove lid. Add pasta and stir well. Seal pot again and select manual and set timer for 5 minutes.
- ❖ Once done, allow to release pressure naturally for 5 minutes then release remaining using quick release. Remove lid. Stir well and serve.

32) Chickpeas Tomato and Red Bell Pasta with Parsley

Preparation Time: 40 minutes

Cooking Time:

Servings: 2

Nutrition: Carbs: 56.4g Protein: 14.47g Fats: 17.7g Calories: 442

Ingredients:

- Pasta: 1 cup cooked
- Chickpeas: 1 cup
- Vegetable broth: 2 cups
- Olive oil: 1 tbsp
- Garlic: 2 cloves minced
- Red bell pepper: ½ cup chopped
- Onion: 1 medium minced
- Tomatoes: 1 cup chopped
- Black pepper: ¼ tsp
- Carrot: 1 diced
- Dried parsley: ½ tsp
- Tomato paste: 1 tbsp

Directions:

- ❖ Cooking Time: pasta as per packet instructions
- ❖ Cooking Time: chickpeas by soaking them overnight and boiling them for two hours on medium heat
- ❖ Take a large saucepan and heat oil on medium flame
- ❖ Add onions and Cooking Time: for 3-4 minutes
- ❖ Add garlic and Cooking Time: for a minute and stir
- ❖ Add tomatoes, bell pepper, carrot, chickpeas, oregano, tomato sauce, and parsley
- ❖ Stir for around a minute or two
- ❖ Add vegetable broth, cover, and boil
- ❖ Simmer for 20-25 minutes until thickened
- ❖ To give a better texture, mash some chickpeas with the back of the spoon
- ❖ Add pasta to the chickpeas soup
- ❖ Season with pepper

33) Cheesy Penna with Red Pepper

Preparation Time: 10 minutes

Cooking Time: 13 minutes

Servings: 6

Nutrition: Calories 459 Fat 10.6 g Carbs 68.1 g Protein 21.3 g

Ingredients:

- 1 lb. whole wheat penne pasta
- 1 tbsp Italian seasoning
- 4 cups vegetable broth
- 1 tbsp garlic, minced
- 1/2 onion, chopped
- 14 oz jar roasted red peppers
- 1 cup feta cheese, crumbled
- 1 tbsp olive oil
- Pepper

Directions:

- ❖ Add roasted pepper into the blender and blend until smooth. Add oil into the inner pot of instant pot and set the pot on sauté mode.
- ❖ Add garlic and onion and sauté for 2-3 minutes. Add blended roasted pepper and sauté for 2 minutes. Add remaining ingredients except feta cheese and stir well.
- ❖ Seal pot with lid and cook on high for 8 minutes. Once done, allow to release pressure naturally for 5 minutes then release remaining using quick release. Remove lid. Top with feta cheese and serve.

34) Milky Brussels Pasta

Preparation Time: 30 minutes

Cooking Time:

Servings: 2

Nutrition: Carbs: 49.75g Protein: 6.75g Fats: 9.65g Calories: 204

Ingredients:
- Macaroni: 1 cup (after cooking
- Brussels sprout: 1 cup halved
- Olive oil: 1 tbsp
- Almond milk: ½ cup
- Flour: 2 tbsp
- Green onion: 1 chopped
- Pepper: as per your taste
- Dried oregano: 2 tbsp

Directions:
- ❖ Cooking Time: pasta as per packet instructions
- ❖ Preheat the oven to 400F
- ❖ In a bowl, add Brussels sprouts and season with pepper and brush with oil
- ❖ Add them to the baking sheet and roast for 20 minutes
- ❖ In a serving tray, spread pasta and top with roasted sprouts
- ❖ In a small pan, heat almond milk and stir in flour
- ❖ Add pasta and sprouts to them and stir to thicken
- ❖ Serve with oregano on top

35) Pasta "Mari e Monti"

Preparation Time: 10 minutes

Cooking Time: 8 minutes

Servings: 6

Nutrition: Calories 346 Fat 11.9g Carbs 31.3g Protein 6.3g

Ingredients:
- 10 oz can tuna, drained
- 15 oz whole wheat rotini pasta
- 4 oz mozzarella cheese, cubed
- 1/2 cup parmesan cheese, grated
- 1 tsp dried basil
- 14 oz can tomato, diced
- 4 cups vegetable broth
- 1 tbsp garlic, minced
- 8 oz mushrooms, sliced
- 2 zucchinis, sliced
- 1 onion, chopped
- 2 tbsp olive oil
- Pepper

Directions:
- ❖ Add oil into the inner pot of instant pot and set the pot on sauté mode. Add mushrooms, zucchini, and onion and sauté until onion is softened. Add garlic and sauté for a minute.
- ❖ Add pasta, basil, tuna, tomatoes, and broth and stir well. Seal pot with lid and cook on high for 4 minutes.
- ❖ Once done, allow to release pressure naturally for 5 minutes then release remaining using quick release. Remove lid. Add remaining ingredients and stir well and serve.

36) Fruity Rice Bowl with Sweet Basil Sauce

Preparation Time: 15 minutes

Cooking Time: 45 minutes

Servings: 4

Nutrition: Calories: 446 Fat: 7.9g Protein: 13.1g Carbs: 85.8g

Ingredients:
Sauce:
- Juice of ¼ lemon
- 2 teaspoons chopped fresh basil
- 1 tablespoon raw honey
- 1 tablespoon extra-virgin olive oil

Rice:
- 1½ cups wild rice
- 2 papayas, peeled, seeded, and diced
- 1 jicama, peeled and shredded
- 1 cup snow peas, julienned
- 2 cups shredded cabbage
- 1 scallion, white and green parts, chopped

Directions:
- ❖ Combine the ingredients for the sauce in a bowl. Stir to mix well. Set aside until ready to use. Pour the wild rice in a saucepan, then pour in enough water to cover. Bring to a boil.
- ❖ Reduce the heat to low, then simmer for 45 minutes or until the wild rice is soft and plump. Drain and transfer to a large serving bowl.
- ❖ Top the rice with papayas, jicama, peas, cabbage, and scallion. Pour the sauce over and stir to mix well before serving.

37) Lettuce Rolls with Beans and Hummus

Preparation Time: 15 minutes

Cooking Time: 10 minutes

Servings: 4

Nutrition: Calories: 211 Fat: 8g Carbs: 28g Protein: 10g

Ingredients:
- 1 tablespoon extra-virgin olive oil
- ½ cup diced red onion (about ¼ onion)
- ¾ cup chopped fresh tomatoes (about 1 medium tomato)
- ¼ teaspoon freshly ground black pepper
- 1 (15-ounce) can cannellini or great northern beans, drained and rinsed
- ¼ cup finely chopped fresh curly parsley
- ½ cup Lemony Garlic Hummus or ½ cup prepared hummus
- 8 romaine lettuce leaves

Directions:
- ❖ In a large skillet over medium heat, heat the oil. Add the onion and cook for 3 minutes, stirring occasionally.
- ❖ Add the tomatoes and pepper and cook for 3 more minutes, stirring occasionally. Add the beans and cook for 3 more minutes, stirring occasionally. Remove from the heat, and mix in the parsley.
- ❖ Spread 1 tablespoon of hummus over each lettuce leaf. Evenly spread the warm bean mixture down the center of each leaf.
- ❖ Fold one side of the lettuce leaf over the filling lengthwise, then fold over the other side to make a wrap and serve.

38) Cauliflower Rice in Chicken Broth

Preparation Time: 15 minutes

Cooking Time: 45 minutes

Servings: 4

Nutrition: Calories: 214 Fat: 3.9g Protein: 7.2g Carbs: 37.9g

Ingredients:

- 1 tablespoon olive oil, plus more for greasing the baking dish
- 1 cup wild rice
- 2 cups low-sodium chicken broth
- 1 sweet onion, chopped
- 2 stalks celery, chopped
- 1 teaspoon minced garlic
- 2 carrots, peeled, halved lengthwise, and sliced
- ½ cauliflower head, cut into small florets
- 1 teaspoon chopped fresh thyme

Directions:

- ❖ Preheat the oven to 350°F (180°C). Line a baking sheet with parchment paper and grease with olive oil.
- ❖ Put the wild rice in a saucepan, then pour in the chicken broth. Bring to a boil. Reduce the heat to low and simmer for 30 minutes or until the rice is plump.
- ❖ Meanwhile, heat the remaining olive oil in an oven-proof skillet over medium-high heat until shimmering.
- ❖ Add the onion, celery, and garlic to the skillet and sauté for 3 minutes or until the onion is translucent.
- ❖ Add the carrots and cauliflower to the skillet and sauté for 5 minutes. Turn off the heat and set aside.
- ❖ Pour the cooked rice in the skillet with the vegetables. Sprinkle with thyme. Set the skillet in the preheated oven and bake for 15 minutes or until the vegetables are soft. Serve immediately.

39) Maple Veggie Macaroni Casserole

Preparation Time: 15 minutes

Cooking Time: 7 hours & 25 minutes

Servings: 5

Nutrition: Calories: 349 Fat: 6.7g Protein: 16.5g Carbs: 59.9g

Ingredients:

- 1 (15-ounce / 425-g) can chickpeas, drained and rinsed
- 1 (28-ounce / 794-g) can diced tomatoes, with the juice
- 1 (6-ounce / 170-g) can no-salt-added tomato paste
- 3 medium carrots, sliced
- 3 cloves garlic, minced
- 1 medium yellow onion, chopped
- 1 cup low-sodium vegetable soup
- ½ teaspoon dried rosemary
- 1 teaspoon dried oregano
- 2 teaspoons maple syrup
- ¼ teaspoon ground black pepper
- ½ pound (227-g) fresh green beans, trimmed and cut into bite-size pieces
- 1 cup macaroni pasta
- 2 ounces (57 g) Parmesan cheese, grated

Directions:

- ❖ Except for the green beans, pasta, and Parmesan cheese, combine all the ingredients in the slow cooker and stir to mix well. Put the slow cooker lid on and cook on low for 7 hours.
- ❖ Fold in the pasta and green beans. Put the lid on and cook on high for 20 minutes or until the vegetable are soft and the pasta is al dente.
- ❖ Pour them in a large serving bowl and spread with Parmesan cheese before serving

40) Red Vinegar Cannellini

Preparation Time: 5 minutes

Cooking Time: 15 minutes

Servings: 6

Nutrition: Calories: 236 Fat: 3g Carbs: 42g Protein: 10g

Ingredients:

- 2 teaspoons extra-virgin olive oil
- ½ cup minced onion (about ¼ onion)
- 1 (12-ounce) can low-sodium tomato paste
- ¼ cup red wine vinegar
- 2 tablespoons honey
- ¼ teaspoon ground cinnamon
- ½ cup water
- 2 (15-ounce) cans cannellini or great northern beans, undrained

Directions:

- ❖ In a medium saucepan over medium heat, heat the oil. Add the onion and cook for 5 minutes, stirring frequently.
- ❖ Add the tomato paste, vinegar, honey, cinnamon, and water, and mix well. Turn the heat to low. Drain and rinse one can of the beans in a colander and add to the saucepan.
- ❖ Pour the entire second can of beans (including the liquid) into the saucepan. Let it cook for 10 minutes, stirring occasionally, and serve.
- ❖ Ingredient tip: Switch up this recipe by making new variations of the homemade ketchup. Instead of the cinnamon, try ¼ teaspoon of smoked paprika and 1 tablespoon of hot sauce. Serve

Chapter 4 -   Side and Salad Recipes

41) Butternut Squash Salad with Pomegranade Dressing

Preparation Time: 10 minutes

Cooking Time: 0 minutes

Servings: 04

Nutrition: Calories 210.6 Fat 10.91 g Carbs 25.6 g Fiber 4.3 g Protein 2.1 g

Ingredients:

- Vegetables:
- 5 cups butternut squash, boiled, peeled, and cubed
- 1 tablespoon coconut oil, melted
- 1 tablespoon coconut sugar
- 1 pinch cayenne pepper
- ½ teaspoon ground cinnamon
- 2 tablespoons maple syrup
- Nuts:
- 1 cup raw pecans
- 2 teaspoons coconut oil
- 1 tablespoon maple syrup
- 1 tablespoon coconut sugar
- 1 pinch cayenne pepper
- ½ teaspoon ground cinnamon
- Pomegranate Dressing:
- ¼ cup pomegranate molasses
- 2 cups mixed greens
- Juice from ½ a medium lemon
- 2 teaspoons olive oil
- Black pepper, to taste
- ½ cup pomegranate arils
- ¼ cup red onion, sliced

Directions:

- ❖ In a salad bowl, add butternut cubes and all the salad ingredients.
- ❖ In a separate bowl, toss all the nuts together.
- ❖ Prepare the dressing by mixing all the dressing ingredients in a different bowl.
- ❖ Add nuts and dressing to the squash and mix well.
- ❖ Serve.

42) Pea Shoot Radish Salad

Preparation Time: 15 minutes

Cooking Time: 5 minutes

Servings: 4-6

Nutrition: Calories: 158 Carbs: 13g Fat: 10g Protein: 4g

Ingredients:

- ¼ cup chopped fresh basil
- ¼ cup extra-virgin olive oil
- ¼ teaspoon ground coriander
- ¼ teaspoon pepper
- 10 radishes, trimmed, halved, and sliced thin
- 1½ ounces (1½ cups) pea shoots
- 2 garlic cloves, minced
- 3 pounds fava beans, shelled (3 cups)
- 3 tablespoons lemon juice

Directions:

- ❖ Bring 4 quarts water to boil in large pot on high heat. In the meantime, fill big container halfway with ice and water.
- ❖ Put in fava beans to boiling water and cook for about sixty seconds. Drain fava beans, move to ice water, and allow to sit until chilled, approximately two minutes.
- ❖ Move fava beans to triple layer of paper towels and dry well. Use a paring knife to make small cut along edge of each bean through waxy sheath, then gently squeeze sheath to release bean; discard sheath.
- ❖ Beat lemon juice, garlic, pepper, and coriander together in a big container. Whisking continuously, slowly drizzle in oil.
- ❖ Put in fava beans, radishes, pea shoots, and basil and gently toss to coat. Serve instantly.

43) Greek Tomato Salad with Feta

Preparation Time: 15 minutes

Cooking Time: 0 minutes

Servings:

Nutrition: Calories: 60 Carbs: 20g Fat: 5g Protein: 0g

Ingredients:

- ¼ cup plain Greek yogurt
- 1 garlic clove, minced
- 1 scallion, sliced thin
- 1 tablespoon extra-virgin olive oil
- 1 tablespoon lemon juice
- 1 tablespoon minced fresh oregano
- 1 teaspoon ground cumin
- 2½ pounds ripe tomatoes, cored and cut into ½-inch-thick wedges
- 3 ounces feta cheese, crumbled (¾ cup)
- Pepper

Directions:

- ❖ Toss tomatoes and allow to drain using a colander set over bowl for fifteen to twenty minutes.
- ❖ Microwave oil, garlic, and cumin in a container until aromatic, approximately half a minute; allow to cool slightly. Move 1 tablespoon tomato liquid to big container; discard remaining liquid.
- ❖ Beat in yogurt, lemon juice, scallion, oregano, and oil mixture until combined. Put in tomatoes and feta and gently toss to coat. Sprinkle pepper to taste. Serve.

44) *Baby Potato Salad with Apple Mustard Dressing*

Preparation Time: 10 minutes

Cooking Time: 0 minutes

Servings: 04

Nutrition: Calories 197 Fat 4 g Carbs 31 g Protein 11 g

Ingredients:

- Potatoes:
- 2 pounds baby yellow potatoes, boiled, peeled, and diced
- 1 pinch black pepper
- 1 tablespoon apple cider vinegar
- 1 cup green onion, diced
- ¼ cup fresh parsley, chopped
- Dressing:
- 2½ tablespoons brown mustard
- 3 cloves garlic, minced
- ¼ teaspoon black pepper
- 3 tablespoons red wine vinegar
- 1 tablespoon apple cider vinegar
- 3 tablespoons olive oil
- ¼ cup dill, chopped

Directions:

- ❖ Combine all the dressing ingredients in a salad bowl.
- ❖ In a salad bowl, toss in all the vegetables, seasonings, and dressing.
- ❖ Mix them well then refrigerate to chill.
- ❖ Serve.

45) *Blood Ricotta Salad*

Preparation Time: 15 minutes

Cooking Time: 0 minutes

Servings: 4-6

Nutrition: Calories: 275 Carbs: 22g Fat: 19g Protein: 5g

Ingredients:

- 2 blood oranges
- 2 ounces (2 cups) baby arugula
- 2 ounces ricotta cheese, shaved
- 2 pounds beets, trimmed
- 2 tablespoons extra-virgin olive oil
- 2 tablespoons sliced almonds, toasted
- 4 teaspoons sherry vinegar
- Pepper

Directions:

- ❖ Place the oven rack in the center of the oven and pre-heat your oven to 400 degrees. Wrap each beet individually in aluminum foil and place in rimmed baking sheet.
- ❖ Roast beets until it is easy to skewer the center of beets with foil removed, forty minutes to one hour.
- ❖ Cautiously open foil packets and allow beets to sit until cool enough to handle. Cautiously rub off beet skins using a paper towel. Slice beets into ½-inch-thick wedges, and, if large, cut in half crosswise.
- ❖ Beat vinegar, ¼ teaspoon salt, and ¼ teaspoon pepper together in a big container. Whisking continuously, slowly drizzle in oil.
- ❖ Put in beets, toss to coat, and allow to cool to room temperature, approximately twenty minutes.
- ❖ Cut away peel and pith from oranges. Quarter oranges, then slice crosswise into ½-inch-thick pieces. Put in oranges and arugula to a container with beets and gently toss to coat.
- ❖ Sprinkle with pepper to taste. Move to serving platter and drizzle with ricotta salata and almonds. Serve.

46) *Exotic Summer Salad*

Preparation Time: 10 minutes

Cooking Time: 0 minutes

Servings: 04

Nutrition: Calories 305 Fat 11.8 g Carbs 34.6 g Protein 7 g

Ingredients:

- Salad:
- 1 head butter lettuce, washed and chopped
- 1½ cups carrot, shredded
- 1¼ cups red cabbage, shredded
- 1 large ripe mango, cubed
- ½ cup fresh cilantro, chopped
- Dressing:
- ⅓ cup creamy peanut butter
- 2½ tablespoons lime juice
- 1½ tablespoons maple syrup
- 2 teaspoon chili garlic sauce
- 3 tablespoons coconut aminos

Directions:

- ❖ Combine all the dressing ingredients in a small bowl.
- ❖ In a salad bowl, toss in all the vegetables, seasonings, and dressing.
- ❖ Mix them well then refrigerate to chill.
- ❖ Serve.

47) Honey Squash Pepitas Salad

Preparation Time: 15 minutes

Cooking Time: 0 minutes

Servings: 4-6

Nutrition: Calories: 385 Carbs: 0g Fat: 6g Protein: 7g

Ingredients:

- ¼ cup extra-virgin olive oil
- 1/3 cup roasted, unsalted pepitas
- ½ cup pomegranate seeds
- ¾ cup fresh parsley leaves
- 1 small shallot, minced
- 1 teaspoon za'atar
- 2 tablespoons honey
- 2 tablespoons lemon juice
- 3 pounds butternut squash, peeled, seeded, and cut into ½-inch pieces (8 cups)
- Pepper

Directions:

- ❖ Place oven rack to lowest position and preheat your oven to 450 degrees. Toss squash with 1 tablespoon oil and sprinkle with pepper.
- ❖ Arrange squash in one layer in rimmed baking sheet and roast until thoroughly browned and tender, 30 to 35 minutes, stirring halfway through roasting. Sprinkle squash with za'atar and allow to cool for about fifteen minutes.
- ❖ Beat shallot, lemon juice, honey together in a big container. Whisking continuously, slowly drizzle in remaining 3 tablespoons oil.
- ❖ Put in squash, parsley, and pepitas and gently toss to coat. Arrange salad on serving platter and drizzle with pomegranate seeds. Serve.

48) Curry Kale Salad with Thaini Dressing

Preparation Time: 10 minutes

Cooking Time: 0 minutes

Servings: 04

Nutrition: Calories 72 Fat 15.4 g Carbs 28.5 g Protein 7.9 g

Ingredients:

- Quinoa:
- ¾ cups quinoa, cooked and drained
- Vegetables:
- 4 large carrots, halved and chopped
- 1 whole beet, sliced
- 2 tablespoons water
- ½ teaspoon curry powder
- 8 cups kale, chopped
- ½ cups cherry tomatoes, chopped
- 1 ripe avocado, cubed
- ¼ cup hemp seeds
- ½ cup sprouts
- Dressing:
- ⅓ cup tahini
- 3 tablespoons lemon juice
- 1-2 tablespoons maple syrup
- ¼ cup water

Directions:

- ❖ Combine all the dressing ingredients in a small bowl.
- ❖ In a salad bowl, toss in all the vegetables, quinoa, and dressing.
- ❖ Mix them well then refrigerate to chill.
- ❖ Serve.

49) Green and Lentil Cauli Salad

Preparation Time: 10 minutes

Cooking Time: 25 minutes

Servings: 04

Nutrition: Calories 212 Fat 7 g Carbs 32.5 g Protein 4 g

Ingredients:

- Cauliflower:
- 1 head cauliflower, florets
- 1½ tablespoons melted coconut oil
- 1½ tablespoons curry powder
- Salad:
- 5 cups mixed greens
- 1 cup cooked lentils
- 1 cup red or green grapes, halved
- Fresh cilantro
- Tahini Dressing:
- 4½ tablespoons green curry paste
- 2 tablespoons tahini
- 2 tablespoons lemon juice
- 1 tablespoon maple syrup
- 1 pinch black pepper
- Water to thin

Directions:

- ❖ Preheat your oven to 400 degrees F.
- ❖ On a greased baking sheet, toss cauliflower with salt, curry powder, and oil.
- ❖ Bake the cauliflower for 25 minutes in the oven.
- ❖ Combine all the dressing ingredients in a small bowl.
- ❖ In a salad bowl, toss in all the vegetables, roasted cauliflower, and dressing.
- ❖ Mix them well then refrigerate to chill.
- ❖ Serve.

50) Creamy Cabbage and Carrots Salad

Preparation Time: 20 minutes

Cooking Time: 10 minutes

Servings: 6

Nutrition: Calories: 192 Fat: 18g Carbs: 7g Protein: 2g

Ingredients:
- 5 cups shredded cabbage
- 2 carrots, shredded
- 1/3 cup chopped fresh flat-leaf parsley
- ½ cup mayonnaise
- ½ cup sour cream
- 3 tablespoons apple cider vinegar
- ½ teaspoon celery seed

Directions:
- ❖ In a large bowl, combine the cabbage, carrots, and parsley. In a small bowl, whisk the mayonnaise, sour cream, vinegar, and celery seed until smooth.
- ❖ Pour the dressing over the vegetables and toss until coated. Transfer to a serving bowl and chill until ready to serve.

51) Roasted Potatoes Green Maple Salad

Preparation Time: 10 minutes

Cooking Time: 10 minutes

Servings: 50

Nutrition: Calories 119 Fat 14 g Carbs 19 g Protein 5g

Ingredients:
- Sweet potato:
- 1 large organic sweet potato, cubed
- 1 tablespoon avocado or coconut oil
- Dressing:
- ¼ cup tahini
- 2 tablespoons lemon juice
- 1 tablespoon maple syrup
- Water
- Salad:
- 5 cups greens of choice
- 1 medium ripe avocado, chopped
- 2 tablespoons hemp seeds

Directions:
- ❖ Preheat your oven to 375 degrees.
- ❖ On a greased baking sheet, toss sweet potato with salt and oil.
- ❖ Bake the potatoes for 20 minutes in the oven, toss halfway through.
- ❖ Combine all the dressing ingredients in a small bowl.
- ❖ In a salad bowl, toss in all the vegetables, roasted potato, and dressing.
- ❖ Mix them well then refrigerate to chill.
- ❖ Serve.

52) Mustard Radish Salad

Preparation Time: 6 minutes

Cooking Time: 0 minutes

Servings: 4

Nutrition: Calories: 87 Fats: 2 g Carbs: 1 g Protein: 2 g

Ingredients:
- 2 tablespoons olive oil
- A pinch of black pepper
- 2 spring onions, chopped
- 3 tablespoons Dijon mustard
- Juice of 1 lime
- ½ cup basil, chopped
- 4 cups romaine lettuce heads, chopped
- 3 radicchios, sliced

Directions:
- ❖ In a salad bowl, mix the lettuce with the spring onions and the other ingredients, toss and serve.

53) Broccoli and Coco Chickpea Salad with Garlic Sauce

Preparation Time: 10 minutes

Cooking Time: 22 minutes

Servings: 06

Nutrition: Calories 231 Fat 20.1 g Carbs 20.1 g Protein 4.6 g

Ingredients:
- Vegetables:
- 1 large sweet potato, peeled and diced
- 1 head broccoli
- 2 tablespoons olive or grapeseed oil
- 1 pinch black pepper
- 1 teaspoon dried dill
- 1 medium red bell pepper
- Chickpeas:
- 1 (15 ouncecan chickpeas, drained
- 1 tablespoon olive or grapeseed oil
- 1 tablespoon tandoori masala spice
- 1 teaspoon coconut sugar
- 1 pinch cayenne pepper
- Garlic dill sauce:
- ⅓ cup hummus
- 3 large cloves garlic, minced
- 1 teaspoon dried dill
- 2 tablespoons lemon juice
- Water

Directions:
- ❖ Preheat your oven to 400 degrees F.
- ❖ In a greased baking sheet, toss sweet potato with oil.
- ❖ Bake the sweet potatoes for 15 minutes in the oven.
- ❖ Toss all chickpea ingredients and spread in a tray.
- ❖ Bake them for 7 minutes in the oven.
- ❖ Combine all the sauce ingredients in a small bowl.
- ❖ In a salad bowl, toss in all the vegetables, roasted potato, chickpeas, and sauce.
- ❖ Mix them well then refrigerate to chill.
- ❖ Serve.

54) Fresh Asparagus and Mustard Fish Salad

Preparation Time: 15 minutes

Cooking Time: 10 minutes

Servings: 8

Nutrition: Calories: 159 Carbs: 7 g Fat: 12.9 g Protein: 6 g

Ingredients:

- 1 lb. fresh asparagus, trimmed and cut into 1-inch pieces
- 1/2 cup pecans,
- 2 heads red leaf lettuce, rinsed and torn
- 1/2 cup frozen green peas, thawed
- 1/4 lb. smoked salmon, cut into 1-inch chunks
- 1/4 cup olive oil
- 2 tablespoons. lemon juice
- 1 teaspoon Dijon mustard
- 1/4 teaspoon pepper

Directions:

- ❖ Boil a pot of water. Stir in asparagus and cook for 5 minutes until tender. Let it drain; set aside. In a skillet, cook the pecans over medium heat for 5 minutes, stirring constantly until lightly toasted.
- ❖ Combine the asparagus, toasted pecans, salmon, peas, and red leaf lettuce and toss in a large bowl.
- ❖ In another bowl, combine lemon juice, pepper, Dijon mustard, and olive oil. You can coat the salad with the dressing or serve it on its side.

55) Red Bell Fennel Salad with Tahini

Preparation Time: 10 minutes

Cooking Time: 20 minutes

Servings: 4

Nutrition: Calories 205 Fat 22.7 g Carbs 26.1 g Protein 5.2 g

Ingredients:

- Fennel:
- 1 bulb fennel fronds, sliced
- 1 tablespoon curry powder
- 1 tablespoon avocado oil
- Salad:
- 5 cups salad greens
- 1 red bell pepper, sliced
- Dressing:
- ¼ cup tahini
- 1½ tablespoons lemon juice
- 1½ teaspoons apple cider vinegar
- 1 tablespoon freshly minced rosemary
- 3 cloves garlic, minced
- 1½ tablespoons coconut aminos
- 5 tablespoons water to thin

Directions:

- ❖ Preheat your oven at 375 degrees F.
- ❖ On a greased baking sheet, toss fennel with curry powder, and oil.
- ❖ Bake the curried fennel for 20 minutes in the oven.
- ❖ Combine all the dressing ingredients in a small bowl.
- ❖ In a salad bowl, toss in all the vegetables, roasted fennel, and dressing.
- ❖ Mix them well then refrigerate to chill.
- ❖ Serve.

56) Chilled Carrot Mix

Preparation Time: 50 minutes

Cooking Time: 0 minutes

Servings: 6

Nutrition: Calories: 159 Fat: 11g Protein: 2g Carbss: 15g

Ingredients:

- ¼ cup extra-virgin olive oil
- Juice of ½ lemon
- 2 tablespoons cider vinegar
- ¼ teaspoon freshly ground black pepper
- Pinch smoked paprika
- Pinch red pepper flakes (optional)
- 1-pound carrots, shredded
- 2 fennel bulbs, trimmed and shredded
- 1/3 cup chopped pitted olives
- 1/3 cup thinly sliced oil-packed sun-dried tomatoes
- ¼ cup chopped fresh flat-leaf parsley

Directions:

- ❖ In a small bowl, whisk together the olive oil, lemon juice, vinegar, black pepper, paprika, and red pepper flakes (if using).
- ❖ In a large bowl, combine the carrots, fennel, olives, and sun-dried tomatoes. Add the dressing and toss well to coat. Chill for 30 minutes, then garnish with the parsley.

57) Cucumber Salad with Red Wine Vinegar

Preparation Time: 15 minutes

Cooking Time: 0 minutes

Servings: 4

Nutrition: Calories: 143 Fat: 14g Protein: 1g Carbs: 4g

Ingredients:

- ¼ cup extra-virgin olive oil
- 1 tablespoon red wine vinegar
- 1 teaspoon dried oregano
- Freshly ground black pepper
- 2 cucumbers, peeled and sliced
- ½ red onion, thinly sliced

Directions:

- ❖ In a small bowl, whisk together the olive oil, vinegar, and oregano. Season with pepper to taste.
- ❖ In a bowl, combine the cucumbers and red onion. Add the dressing and toss well to coat.

58) Zucchini and Potato Salad with Coco Dressing

Preparation Time: 10 minutes

Cooking Time: 20 minutes

Servings: 04

Nutrition: Calories 201 Fat 8.9 g Carbs 24.7 g Protein 15.3 g

Ingredients:

- Roasted vegetables:
- 1 medium zucchini, chopped
- 1 medium sweet potato, chopped
- 1 cup red cabbage, chopped
- 1 tablespoon melted coconut oil
- ½ teaspoon curry powder
- Dressing:
- ⅓ cup tahini
- ½ teaspoon garlic powder
- 1 tablespoon coconut aminos
- 1 large clove garlic, minced
- ¼ cup water
- Salad:
- 6 cups mixed greens
- 4 small radishes, sliced
- 3 tablespoons hemp seeds
- 2 tablespoons lemon juice
- ½ ripe avocado, to garnish
- 2 tablespoons vegan feta cheese, crumbled
- Pomegranate seeds, to garnish
- Pecans, to garnish

Directions:

- ❖ Preheat your oven at 375 degrees F.
- ❖ On a greased baking sheet, toss zucchini, sweet potato, and red cabbage with curry powder, and oil.
- ❖ Bake the zucchini cabbage mixture for 20 minutes in the oven.
- ❖ Combine all the dressing ingredients in a small bowl.
- ❖ In a salad bowl, toss in all the vegetables, roasted vegetables, and dressing.
- ❖ Mix them well then refrigerate to chill.
- ❖ Garnish with feta cheese, pecans, pomegranate seeds and avocado.
- ❖ Serve.

59) Bulgur Mixture with Fresh Mint

Preparation Time: 15 minutes

Cooking Time: 20 minutes

Servings: 4

Nutrition: Calories: 271 Fat: 14g Protein: 6g Carbs: 34g

Ingredients:

- 1 cup bulgur
- 4 plum tomatoes, diced, juices reserved
- 2 cups finely chopped fresh flat-leaf parsley
- 4 scallions, chopped
- ¼ cup extra-virgin olive oil
- Juice of 2 lemons
- 2 tablespoons finely chopped fresh mint
- ¼ teaspoon freshly ground black pepper

Directions:

- ❖ In a saucepan, prepare the bulgur according to package directions. Drain thoroughly, transfer to a large bowl, and set aside to cool. Once cool, add the tomatoes with their juices, parsley, and scallions.
- ❖ In a small bowl, whisk together the olive oil, lemon juice, mint and pepper. Pour the dressing over the bulgur mixture and toss to coat.

60) Cheesy Macadamia Squash Salad

Preparation Time: 10 minutes

Cooking Time: 20 minutes

Servings: 04

Nutrition: Calories 119 Fat 14 g Carbs 19 g Protein 5g

Ingredients:

- Squash:
- 1 medium acorn squash, peeled and cubed
- 1 tablespoon avocado oil
- 1 pinch black pepper
- Dressing:
- 1 cup balsamic vinegar
- Salad:
- ¼ cup macadamia nut cheese
- 2 tablespoons roasted pumpkin seeds
- 5 cups arugula
- 2 tablespoons dried currants

Directions:

- ❖ Preheat your oven to 425 degrees F.
- ❖ On a greased baking sheet, toss squash with salt, black pepper, and oil.
- ❖ Bake the seasoned squash for 20 minutes in the oven.
- ❖ Combine all the dressing ingredients in a small bowl.
- ❖ In a salad bowl, toss in the squash, salad ingredients, and dressing.
- ❖ Mix them well then refrigerate to chill.
- ❖ Serve.

Chapter 5 -   Main Recipes

61) Tex-Mex Lettuce Bowl

Preparation Time: 5minutes

Cooking Time: 10minutes

Servings: 4

Nutrition: Calories: 263, Fat: 26.4g, Carbs:4g, Protein:4g,

Ingredients:

- 2 tbsp Tex-Mex seasoning
- 1 small iceberg lettuce, chopped
- 2 large tomatoes, deseeded and chopped
- 2 avocados, halved, pitted, and chopped
- 1 green bell pepper, deseeded and thinly sliced
- 1 yellow onion, thinly sliced
- 4 tbsp fresh cilantro leaves
- ½ cup shredded dairy- free parmesan cheese blend
- 1 cup plain unsweetened yogurt

Directions:

- ❖ Heat the olive oil in a medium skillet over medium heat, season the tofu with black pepper, and Tex-Mex seasoning. Fry in the oil on both sides until golden and cooked, 5 to 10 minutes. Transfer to a plate.
- ❖ Divide the lettuce into 4 serving bowls, share the tofu on top, and add the tomatoes, avocados, bell pepper, onion, cilantro, and cheese.
- ❖ Top with dollops of plain yogurt and serve immediately

62) Double Chicken Pesto Cream

Preparation Time: 10 minutes

Cooking Time: 12 minutes

Servings: 4

Nutrition: Calories 341 Fat 15.2 g Carbs 4.4 g Protein 43.8 g

Ingredients:

- 4 chicken breasts, skinless and boneless
- 1 tbsp basil pesto
- 1 1/2 tbsp cornstarch
- 1/4 cup roasted red peppers, chopped
- 1/3 cup heavy cream
- 1 tsp Italian seasoning
- 1 tsp garlic, minced
- 1 cup chicken broth
- Pepper

Directions:

- ❖ Add chicken into the instant pot. Season chicken with Italian seasoning and pepper. Sprinkle with garlic. Pour broth over chicken. Seal pot with lid and cook on high for 8 minutes.
- ❖ Once done, allow to release pressure naturally for 5 minutes then release remaining using quick release. Remove lid. Transfer chicken on a plate and clean the instant pot.
- ❖ Set instant pot on sauté mode. Add heavy cream, pesto, cornstarch, and red pepper to the pot and stir well and cook for 3-4 minutes.
- ❖ Return chicken to the pot and coat well with the sauce. Serve and enjoy.

63) Italian Spicy Tofurella

Preparation Time: 10minutes

Cooking Time: 35minutes

Servings: 4

Nutrition: Calories: 140, Fat: 13.2g, Carbs:2g, Protein:3g,

Ingredients:

- 1½ lb tofu, halved lengthwise
- Ground black pepper to taste
- 2 eggs
- 2 tbsp Italian seasoning
- 1 pinch red chili flakes
- ½ cup sliced Pecorino Romano cheese
- ¼ cup fresh parsley, chopped
- 4 tbsp butter
- 2 garlic cloves, minced
- 2 cups crushed tomatoes
- 1 tbsp dried basil
- ½ lb sliced mozzarella cheese

Directions:

- ❖ Preheat the oven to 400 F and grease a baking dish with cooking spray. Set aside.
- ❖ Season the tofu with black pepper; set aside.
- ❖ In a medium bowl, whisk the eggs with the Italian seasoning, and red chili flakes. In a plate, combine the Pecorino Romano cheese with parsley.
- ❖ Melt the butter in a medium skillet over medium heat.
- ❖ Quickly dip the tofu in the egg mixture and then dredge generously in the cheese mixture. Place in the butter and fry on both sides until the cheese melts and is golden brown, 8 to 10 minutes. Place on a plate and set aside.
- ❖ Sauté the garlic in the same pan and mix in the tomatoes. Top with the basil and black pepper, and Cooking Time: for 5 to 10 minutes. Pour the sauce into the baking dish.
- ❖ Lay the tofu pieces in the sauce and top with the mozzarella cheese. Bake in the oven for 10 to 15 minutes or until the cheese melts completely.
- ❖ Remove the dish and serve with leafy green salad.

64) Simple Chicken Bell Pepper

Preparation Time: 10 minutes

Cooking Time: 25 minutes

Servings: 4

Nutrition: Calories 254 Fat 9.9 g Carbs 4.6 g Protein 34.6 g

Ingredients:

- 3 chicken breasts, skinless, boneless, and sliced
- 1 tsp garlic, minced
- 1 tbsp Italian seasoning
- 2 cups chicken broth
- 1 bell pepper, sliced
- 1/2 onion, sliced
- Pepper

Directions:

- ❖ Add chicken into the instant pot and top with remaining ingredients. Seal pot with lid and cook on high for 25 minutes. Once done, release pressure using quick release. Remove lid.
- ❖ Remove chicken from pot and shred using a fork. Return shredded chicken to the pot and stir well. Serve over cooked whole grain pasta and top with cheese.

65) American Yellow Cheddar Tempeh

Preparation Time: 10minutes

Cooking Time: 20minutes

Servings: 4

Nutrition: Calories:132, Total Fat:11.5g, Carbs:7g, Protein:1g

Ingredients:

- 1 Tempeh, shredded
- 1/3 cup vegan mayonnaise
- 8 oz dairy- free cream cheese (vegan
- 1 yellow onion, sliced
- 1 yellow bell pepper, deseeded and chopped
- 2 tbsp taco seasoning
- ½ cup shredded cheddar cheese
- Ground black pepper to taste

Directions:

- ❖ Preheat the oven to 400 F and grease a baking dish with cooking spray.
- ❖ Into the dish, put the tempeh, mayonnaise, cashew cream, onion, bell pepper, taco seasoning, and two-thirds of the cheese, salt, and black pepper. Mix the Ingredients and top with the remaining cheese.
- ❖ Bake in the oven for 15 to 20 minutes or until the cheese melts and is golden brown.
- ❖ Remove the dish, plate, and serve with lettuce leaves.

66) Latin Flag Rice

Preparation Time: 10 minutes

Cooking Time: 15 minutes

Servings: 6

Nutrition: Calories 494 Fat 11.3 g Carbs 61.4 g Protein 34.2 g

Ingredients:

- 1 lb. chicken breasts, skinless, boneless, and cut into chunks
- 14 oz can cannellini beans, rinsed and drained
- 4 cups chicken broth
- 2 cups brown rice
- 1 tbsp Italian seasoning
- 1 small onion, chopped
- 1 tbsp garlic, chopped
- 1 tbsp olive oil
- Pepper

Directions:

- ❖ Add oil into the inner pot of instant pot and set the pot on sauté mode. Add garlic and onion and sauté for 3 minutes. Add remaining ingredients and stir everything well.
- ❖ Seal pot with a lid and select manual and set timer for 12 minutes. Once done, release pressure using quick release. Remove lid. Stir well and serve.

67) Creamy Kale Broccoli with Parmesan Cheese

Preparation Time: 10minutes

Cooking Time: 15minutes

Servings: 4

Nutrition: Calories: 193, Fat: 20.1g, Carbs:3g, Protein:1g,

Ingredients:

- 6 slices tempeh, chopped
- 2 tbsp butter
- 4 tofu, cut into 1-inch cubes
- Ground black pepper to taste
- 4 garlic cloves, minced
- 1 cup baby kale, chopped
- 1 ½ cups full- fat heavy creaminutes
- 1 medium head broccoli, cut into florets
- ¼ cup shredded parmesan cheese

Directions:

- ❖ Put the tempeh in a medium skillet over medium heat and fry until crispy and brown, 5 minutes. Spoon onto a plate and set aside.
- ❖ Melt the butter in the same skillet, season the tofu with black pepper, and Cooking Time: on both sides until goldern- brown. Spoon onto the tempeh's plate and set aside.
- ❖ Add the garlic to the skillet, sauté for 1 minute.
- ❖ Mix in the full- fat heavy cream, tofu, and tempeh, and kale, allow simmering for 5 minutes or until the sauce thickens.
- ❖ Meanwhile, pour the broccoli into a large safe-microwave bowl, sprinkle with some water, season with black pepper, and microwave for 2 minutes or until the broccoli softens.
- ❖ Spoon the broccoli into the sauce, top with the parmesan cheese, stir and Cooking Time: until the cheese melts. Turn the heat off.
- ❖ Spoon the mixture into a serving platter and serve warm.

68) Red Cherry Asparagus Chicken

Preparation Time: 10 minutes

Cooking Time: 25 minutes

Servings: 4

Nutrition: Calories 459 Fat 20 g Carbs 14.9 g Protein 9.2 g

Ingredients:

- 1 1/2 lb. chicken thighs, skinless, boneless, and cut into pieces
- 1/2 cup chicken broth
- 1/4 cup fresh parsley, chopped
- 2 cups cherry tomatoes, halved
- 1 cup basil pesto
- 3/4 lb. asparagus, trimmed and cut in half
- 2/3 cup sun-dried tomatoes, drained and chopped
- 2 tbsp olive oil
- Pepper

Directions:

- ❖ Add oil into the inner pot of instant pot and set the pot on sauté mode. Add chicken and sauté for 5 minutes. Add remaining ingredients except for tomatoes and stir well.
- ❖ Seal pot with a lid and select manual and set timer for 15 minutes. Once done, release pressure using quick release. Remove lid.
- ❖ Add tomatoes and stir well. Again, seal the pot and select manual and set timer for 5 minutes. Release pressure using quick release. Remove lid. Stir well and serve.

69) Baked Bell Peppers with Yogurt Topping

Preparation Time: 15 minutes

Cooking Time: 41 minutes

Servings: 6

Nutrition: Calories: 251, **Fat:** 22.5g, **Carbs:** 13g, **Protein:** 3g,

Ingredients:

- 6 yellow bell peppers, halved and deseeded
- 1 ½ tbsp olive oil
- Ground black pepper to taste
- 3 tbsp butter
- 3 garlic cloves, minced
- ½ white onion, chopped
- 2 lbs. ground tempeh
- 3 tsp taco seasoning
- 1 cup riced broccoli
- ¼ cup grated cheddar cheese
- Plain unsweetened yogurt for serving

Directions:

- ❖ Preheat the oven to 400 F and grease a baking dish with cooking spray. Set aside.
- ❖ Drizzle the bell peppers with the olive oil. Set aside.
- ❖ Melt the butter in a large skillet and sauté the garlic and onion for 3 minutes. Stir in the tempeh, taco seasoning, salt, and black pepper. Cooking Time: until the meat is no longer pink, 8 minutes.
- ❖ Mix in the broccoli until adequately incorporated. Turn the heat off.
- ❖ Spoon the mixture into the peppers, top with the cheddar cheese, and place the peppers in the baking dish. Bake in the oven until the cheese melts and is bubbly, 30 minutes.
- ❖ Remove the dish from the oven and plate the peppers. Top with the palin yogurt and serve warm.

70) Coriander Shrimp with Lemon Juice

Preparation Time: 20 minutes

Cooking Time: 10 minutes

Servings: 4

Nutrition: Calories: 225 **Fat:** 12g **Protein:** 28g **Carbs:** 5g

Ingredients:

- 1/3 cup lemon juice
- 4 garlic cloves
- 1 cup fresh cilantro leaves
- ½ teaspoon ground coriander
- 3 tablespoons extra-virgin olive oil
- 1½ pounds (680 g) large shrimp (21 to 25), deveined and shells removed

Directions:

- ❖ In a food processor, pulse the lemon juice, garlic, cilantro, coriander and olive oil 10 times. Put the shrimp in a bowl or plastic zip-top bag, pour in the cilantro marinade, and let sit for 15 minutes.
- ❖ Preheat a skillet on high heat. Put the shrimp and marinade in the skillet. Cook the shrimp for 3 minutes on each side. Serve warm.

71) Veggie Bacon and Tofu Rolls

Preparation Time: 5 minutes

Cooking Time: 20 minutes

Servings: 4

Nutrition: Calories: 260, **Fat:** 24.7g, **Carbs:** 4g, **Protein:** 6g

Ingredients:

- For the bacon wrapped tofu:
- 4 tofu
- 8 slices vegan bacon
- Black pepper to taste
- 2 tbsp olive oil
- For the buttered spinach:
- 2 tbsp butter
- 1 lb spinach
- 4 garlic cloves

Directions:

- ❖ For the bacon wrapped tofu:
- ❖ Preheat the oven to 450 F.
- ❖ Wrap each tofu with two vegan bacon slices, season with black pepper, and place on the baking sheet. Drizzle with the olive oil and bake in the oven for 15 minutes or until the vegan bacon browns and the tofu cooks within.
- ❖ For the buttered spinach:
- ❖ Meanwhile, melt the butter in a large skillet, add and sauté the spinach and garlic until the leaves wilt, 5 minutes. Season with black pepper.
- ❖ Remove the tofu from the oven and serve with the buttered spinach.

72) Delicious Italian "Risotto di Mare"

Preparation Time: 15 minutes

Cooking Time: 30 minutes

Servings: 4

Nutrition: Calories: 460 Fat: 12g Protein: 24g Carbs: 64g

Ingredients:

- 6 cups vegetable broth
- 3 tablespoons extra-virgin olive oil
- 1 large onion, chopped
- 3 cloves garlic, minced
- ½ teaspoon saffron threads
- 1½ cups arborio rice
- 8 ounces (227 g) shrimp (21 to 25), peeled and deveined
- 8 ounces (227 g) scallops

Directions:

- ❖ In a large saucepan over medium heat, bring the broth to a low simmer. In a large skillet over medium heat, cook the olive oil, onion, garlic, and saffron for 3 minutes.
- ❖ Add the rice, salt, and 1 cup of the broth to the skillet. Stir the ingredients together and cook over low heat until most of the liquid is absorbed.
- ❖ Repeat steps with broth, adding ½ cup of broth at a time, and cook until all but ½ cup of the broth is absorbed.
- ❖ Add the shrimp and scallops when you stir in the final ½ cup of broth. Cover and let cook for 10 minutes. Serve warm.

73) Healthy Mushroom Kebab

Preparation Time: 15 minutes

Cooking Time: 12 minutes

Servings: 4

Nutrition: Calories 58 Fat 2 g Carbs 9 g Protein 2 g

Ingredients:

- 2 cloves garlic, minced
- ¼ cup balsamic vinegar
- ¼ cup olive oil
- 1 tablespoon Italian seasoning
- Pepper to taste
- 1 onion, sliced into quarters
- 12 medium mushrooms
- 16 cherry tomatoes
- 1 zucchini, sliced into rounds
- 1 cup tofu, cubed
- 4 cups cauliflower rice

Directions:

- ❖ In a bowl, mix the garlic, vinegar, oil, Italian seasoning and pepper.
- ❖ Toss the vegetable slices and tofu in the mixture.
- ❖ Marinate for 1 hour.
- ❖ Thread into 8 skewers and grill for 12 minutes, turning once or twice.
- ❖ Add cauliflower rice into 4 food containers.
- ❖ Add 2 kebab skewers on top of each container of cauliflower rice.
- ❖ Reheat kebabs in the grill before serving.

74) Lobster Calamari and Shrimp Paella

Preparation Time: 15 minutes

Cooking Time: 20 minutes

Servings: 4

Nutrition: Calories: 632 Fat: 20g Protein: 34g Carbs: 71g

Ingredients:

- ¼ cup plus 1 tablespoon extra-virgin olive oil
- 1 large onion, finely chopped
- 2 tomatoes, peeled and chopped
- 1½ tablespoons garlic powder
- 1½ cups medium-grain Spanish paella rice or arborio rice
- 2 carrots, finely diced
- 1 tablespoon sweet paprika
- 8 ounces (227 g) lobster meat or canned crab
- ½ cup frozen peas
- 3 cups chicken stock, plus more if needed
- 1 cup dry white wine
- 6 jumbo shrimp, unpeeled
- ⅓ pound (136 g) calamari rings
- 1 lemon, halved

Directions:

- ❖ In a large sauté pan or skillet (16-inch is ideal), heat the oil over medium heat until small bubbles start to escape from oil.
- ❖ Add the onion and cook for about 3 minutes, until fragrant, then add tomatoes and garlic powder. Cook for 5 to 10 minutes, until the tomatoes are reduced by half and the consistency is sticky.
- ❖ Stir in the rice, carrots, paprika, lobster, and peas and mix well. In a pot or microwave-safe bowl, heat the chicken stock to almost boiling, then add it to the rice mixture. Bring to a simmer, then add the wine.
- ❖ Smooth out the rice in the bottom of the pan. Cover and cook on low for 10 minutes, mixing occasionally, to prevent burning.
- ❖ Top the rice with the shrimp, cover, and cook for 5 more minutes. Add additional broth to the pan if the rice looks dried out.
- ❖ Right before removing the skillet from the heat, add the calamari rings. Toss the ingredients frequently.
- ❖ In about 2 minutes, the rings will look opaque. Remove the pan from the heat immediately—you don't want the paella to overcook). Squeeze fresh lemon juice over the dish.

75) Tamari Carrot And Radish with Cilantro

Preparation Time: 10 minutes

Cooking Time: 0 minute

Servings: 4

Nutrition: Calories 98 Fat 8 g Carbs 6 g Protein 2 g

Ingredients:

- 2 tablespoons sesame oil, toasted
- 3 tablespoons rice vinegar
- ½ teaspoon sugar
- 2 tablespoons low sodium tamari
- 1 cup carrots, sliced into strips
- 2 cups radishes, sliced
- 2 tablespoons fresh cilantro, chopped
- 2 teaspoons sesame seeds, toasted

Directions:

- ❖ Mix the oil, vinegar, sugar and tamari in a bowl.
- ❖ Add the carrots, radishes and cilantro.
- ❖ Toss to coat evenly.
- ❖ Let sit for 10 minutes.
- ❖ Transfer to a food container.

76) Crispistachio Whitefish

Preparation Time: 10 minutes

Cooking Time: 20 minutes

Servings: 2

Nutrition: Calories: 185, Carbs: 23.8 g, Protein: 10.1 g, Fat: 5.2 g

Ingredients:

- ¼ cup shelled pistachios
- 1 tablespoon fresh parsley
- 1 tablespoon grated Parmesan cheese
- 1 tablespoon panko bread crumbs
- 2 tablespoons olive oil
- 10 ounces skinless whitefish (1 large piece or 2 smaller ones)

Directions:

- ❖ Preheat the oven to 350°F and set the rack to the middle position. Line a sheet pan with foil or parchment paper.
- ❖ Combine all of the ingredients except the fish in a mini food processor, and pulse until the nuts are finely ground.
- ❖ Alternatively, you can mince the nuts with a chef's knife and combine the ingredients by hand in a small bowl.
- ❖ Place the fish on the sheet pan. Spread the nut mixture evenly over the fish and pat it down lightly.
- ❖ Bake the fish for 20 to 30 minutes, depending on the thickness, until it flakes easily with a fork.
- ❖ Keep in mind that a thicker cut of fish takes a bit longer to bake. You'll know it's done when it's opaque, flakes apart easily with a fork, or reaches an internal temperature of 145°F

77) Lemony Baked Vegetables

Preparation Time: 15 minutes

Cooking Time: 20 minutes

Servings: 5

Nutrition: Calories 52 Fat 3 g Carbs 5 g Protein 2 g

Ingredients:

- 2 cloves garlic, sliced
- 1 ½ cups broccoli florets
- 1 ½ cups cauliflower florets
- 1 tablespoon olive oil
- 1 teaspoon dried oregano, crushed
- ¾ cup zucchini, diced
- ¾ cup red bell pepper, diced
- 2 teaspoons lemon zest

Directions:

- ❖ Preheat your oven to 425 degrees F.
- ❖ In a baking pan, add the garlic, broccoli and cauliflower.
- ❖ Toss in oil and season with oregano.
- ❖ Roast in the oven for 10 minutes.
- ❖ Add the zucchini and bell pepper to the pan.
- ❖ Stir well.
- ❖ Roast for another 10 minutes.
- ❖ Sprinkle lemon zest on top before serving.
- ❖ Transfer to a food container and reheat before serving.

78) Salmon Paprika Sticks

Preparation Time: 10 minutes

Cooking Time: 15 minutes

Servings: 2

Nutrition: 119 Cal, 3.4g fat, 9.3g carbs, 13.5g protein.

Ingredients:

- ½ cup of flour
- 1 beaten egg
- 1 cup of flour
- ½ cup of parmesan cheese
- ½ cup of bread crumbs.
- Zest of 1 lemon juice
- Parsley
- 1 teaspoon of black pepper
- 1 tablespoon of sweet paprika
- 1 teaspoon of oregano
- 1 ½ lb. of salmon
- Extra virgin olive oil

Directions:

- ❖ Preheat your oven to about 450 degrees F. Get a bowl, dry your salmon.
- ❖ Then chop into small sizes of 1½ inch length each. Get a bowl and mix black pepper with oregano.
- ❖ Add paprika to the mixture and blend it. Then spice the fish stick with the mixture you have just made. Get another dish and pour your flours.
- ❖ You will need a different bowl again to pour your egg wash into. Pick yet the fourth dish, mix your breadcrumb with your parmesan and add lemon zest to the mixture.
- ❖ Return to the fish sticks and dip each fish into flour such that both sides are coated with flour. As you dip each fish into flour, take it out and dip it into egg wash and lastly, dip it in the breadcrumb mixture.
- ❖ Do this for all fish sticks and arrange on a baking sheet. Ensure you oil the baking sheet before arranging the stick thereon and drizzle the top of the fish sticks with extra virgin olive oil.
- ❖ Caution: allow excess flours to fall off a fish before dipping it into other ingredients.
- ❖ Also ensure that you do not let the coating peel while you add extra virgin olive oil on top of the fishes.
- ❖ Fix the baking sheet in the middle of the oven and allow it to cook for 13 min. By then, the fishes should be golden brown and you can collect them from the oven, and you can serve immediately.
- ❖ Top it with your lemon zest, parsley and fresh lemon juice.

79) Splash Beans and Potatoes with Tamari Sauce

Preparation Time:

Cooking Time: 10 minutes

Servings: 4

Nutrition: Calories 232 Fat 2.1g Carbohydrate 44.2g

Ingredients:

- 4 whole-wheat tortillas
- 2 potatoes, boiled, cubed
- 200g refried beans
- 1 teaspoon chili powder
- ½ teaspoon dried oregano
- ¼ teaspoon garlic powder
- 120g spinach
- 1 onion, thinly sliced
- 2 cloves garlic, minced
- 30ml tamari sauce
- 45g nutritional yeast
- Pepper, to taste

Directions:

- ❖ Heat a splash of olive oil in a skillet.
- ❖ Add onion and Cooking Time: over medium heat for 10 minutes, or until the onion is caramelized.
- ❖ Add the garlic and Cooking Time: 1 minute.
- ❖ Add spinach and toss gently.
- ❖ Add tamari sauce and Cooking Time: 1 minutes.
- ❖ Reheat the refried beans with nutritional yeast, chili, oregano, and garlic powder, in a microwave, on high for 1 minute.
- ❖ Mash the potatoes and spread over tortilla.
- ❖ Top the mashed potatoes with spinach mixture and refried beans.
- ❖ Season to taste and place another tortilla on top.
- ❖ Heat large skillet over medium-high heat.
- ❖ Heat the tortilla until crispy. Flip and heat the other side.
- ❖ Cut the tortilla in half and serve.

80) *Sliced Cuttlefish in Robola Wine*

Preparation Time: 10 minutes

Cooking Time: 10 minutes

Servings: 2

Nutrition: Calories: 308, Fats: 18.1g, Carbs: 8g, Protein: 25.6g

Ingredients:

- 2-lbs fresh cuttlefish
- ½-cup olive oil
- 1-pc large onion, finely chopped
- 1-cup of Robola white wine
- ¼-cup lukewarm water
- 1-pc bay leaf
- ½-bunch parsley, chopped
- 4-pcs tomatoes, grated
- Pepper

Directions:

- ❖ Take out the hard centerpiece of cartilage (cuttlebone), the bag of ink, and the intestines from the cuttlefish.
- ❖ Wash the cleaned cuttlefish with running water. Slice it into small pieces, and drain excess water.
- ❖ Heat the oil in a saucepan placed over medium-high heat and sauté the onion for 3 minutes until tender.
- ❖ Add the sliced cuttlefish and pour in the white wine. Cook for 5 minutes until it simmers.
- ❖ Pour in the water, and add the tomatoes, bay leaf, parsley, tomatoes, and pepper. Simmer the mixture over low heat until the cuttlefish slices are tender and left with their thick sauce. Serve them warm with rice.
- ❖ Be careful not to overcook the cuttlefish as its texture becomes very hard. A safe rule of thumb is grilling the cuttlefish over a ragingly hot fire for 3 minutes before using it in any recipe.

Chapter 6 -   Soup Recipes

81) Ginger Mushroom Soup with Walnuts Topping

Preparation Time: 10 minutes

Cooking Time: 14 minutes

Servings: 4

Nutrition: Calories 923, Fat 8.59g, Carbs 12.23g, Protein 23.48g

Ingredients:

- 1 tbsp olive oil
- 2/3 cup sliced white button mushrooms
- 1 large white onion, finely chopped
- 1 garlic clove, minced
- 1 tsp ginger puree
- 1 cup vegetable broth
- 2 turnips, peeled and chopped
- Freshly ground black pepper to taste
- 2 (14 ozsilken tofu, drained and rinsed
- 2 cups unsweetened almond milk
- 1 tbsp freshly chopped oregano
- 1 tbsp freshly chopped parsley to garnish
- 1 tbsp chopped walnuts for topping

Directions:

- ❖ Over medium fire, heat olive oil in a large saucepan and Cooking Time: mushrooms until softened, 5 minutes. Remove onto a plate and set aside.
- ❖ Add and sauté onion, garlic, and ginger puree until fragrant and soft.
- ❖ Pour in vegetable broth, turnips, and black pepper. Cooking Time: until turnips soften, 6 minutes.
- ❖ Add silken tofu and using an immersion blender, puree ingredients until very smooth.
- ❖ Stir in mushrooms and simmer until mushrooms heat through, 2 to 3 minutes. Make sure to stir soup frequently to prevent tofu from curdling.
- ❖ Add almond milk and adjust taste with black pepper. Stir in oregano and dish soup.
- ❖ Garnish with parsley and serve with soy chorizo chips.

82) Ditalini in Chicken Broth with Eggs

Preparation Time: 15 minutes

Cooking Time: 0 minutes

Servings: 2

Nutrition: Calories: 161 Protein: 10 g Fat: 2 g Carbs: 65 g

Ingredients:

- 4 ounces ditalini pasta
- 4 cups fat-free and low-sodium chicken broth
- 2 large whole eggs
- ½ cup fresh lemon juice
- 4 tablespoons chopped fresh parsley
- 1 lemon, thinly sliced for garnish
- Freshly ground pepper to taste

Directions:

- ❖ Place medium saucepan on medium-high heat. Add chicken broth to it and bring it to a boil, stirring it a couple of times.
- ❖ Bring down the heat to low and allow the broth to simmer for about 5 minutes. Take the saucepan off the heat.
- ❖ Take a bowl and add the eggs into it. Beat them well, add the lemon juice, and beat the eggs again
- ❖ Use a ladle to transfer a single serving of the chicken broth into the egg bowl. Mix them well and then transfer the entire contents of the bowl into the saucepan.
- ❖ Heat the soup while ensuring that the heat is still at low. Keep an eye out on the eggs because they tend to curdle and you need to prevent that from happening by gently stirring the soup.
- ❖ Add pepper to taste, if preferred.
- ❖ Serve hot and garnish with lemon slices and parsley.

83) Aparagus and Beans Soup with Parmesan Cheese

Preparation Time: 8 minutes

Cooking Time: 12 minutes

Servings: 4

Nutrition: Calories 196, Fat 11.9g, Carbs 10.02g, Protein 3g

Ingredients:

- 4 cups vegetable stock
- 3 cups green beans, chopped
- 2 cups asparagus, chopped
- 1 cup pearl onions, peeled and halved
- 2 cups seaweed mix (or spinach
- 1 tbsp garlic powder
- Freshly ground white pepper to taste
- 2 cups grated Parmesan cheese, for serving

Directions:

- ❖ In a large pot, add vegetable stock, green beans, asparagus, and pearl onions. Season with garlic powder and white pepper.
- ❖ Cover pot and Cooking Time: over low heat until vegetables soften, 10 minutes.
- ❖ Stir in seaweed mix and adjust taste with white pepper.
- ❖ Dish into serving bowls and top with plenty of Parmesan cheese.
- ❖ Serve with low carb bread.

84) Low Fat Milky Green Soup

Preparation Time: 10 minutes

Cooking Time: 30 minutes

Servings: 2

Nutrition: Calories: 163 calories Protein: 4 g Fat: 8 g Carbs: 15 g

Ingredients:

- 5 ounces fresh green beans, thinly sliced
- 8 ounces fresh Brussels sprouts, sliced
- 5 cups low-sodium, fat-free vegetable broth
- 1½ cups frozen peas, defrosted
- 4 tablespoons olive oil
- 1 white onion, chopped
- 1 tablespoon freshly squeezed lemon juice
- 4 cloves fresh garlic, minced
- 1 large leek, slice both white parts and sliced green parts thinly but keep them separate
- 1 teaspoon ground coriander
- 1 cup low-fat milk
- Freshly ground pepper to taste
- Croutons for garnish

Directions:

- ❖ Take out a large skillet and place it over low heat. Add the olive oil and allow the oil to heat up slightly.
- ❖ Add onion and garlic. Cook them until they turn fragrant and soft. Make sure that you do not allow them to turn brown.
- ❖ Add the green parts of the Brussels sprouts, leek, and green beans to the skillet. Add the broth and mix the ingredients well. Bring the broth to a boil. When it starts boiling, lower the heat and let simmer for about 12 minutes.
- ❖ Add lemon juice, peas, and coriander. Let the broth continue to simmer for another 10 minutes, or until the vegetables become tender.
- ❖ Remove the broth mixture from heat and allow it to cool slightly. Transfer the mixture to a blender and pulse until they turn smooth.
- ❖ Take out a saucepan and add the white parts of leek. Add the blended mixture into the saucepan. Place the saucepan over medium high heat and allow the soup to boil. Reduce the heat to low and allow the soup to simmer for about 5 minutes
- ❖ Take out another bowl and add flour and milk. Whisk them until they turn smooth.
- ❖ Add pepper to taste, if preferred.

85) Coconut Cauliflower and Onion Soup

Preparation Time: 10 minutes

Cooking Time: 4 hours 5 minutes

Servings: 4

Nutrition: Calories 119 Fat 14 g Carbs 19 g Protein 5g

Ingredients:

- 2 tablespoons olive oil
- 1½ cups sweet white onion, chopped
- 2 large cloves of garlic, chopped
- 1 head cauliflower, cut into florets
- 1 cup coconut milk
- 1 cup filtered water
- 1 teaspoon vegetable stock paste
- 2 tablespoons nutritional yeast
- Dash of olive oil
- Fresh cracked pepper
- Parsley, to serve

Directions:

- ❖ Add olive oil and onion to a slow cooker.
- ❖ Sauté for 5 minutes then add the rest of the ingredients.
- ❖ Put on the slow cooker's lid and Cooking Time: for 4 hours on low heat.
- ❖ Once done, blend the soup with a hand blender.
- ❖ Garnish with parsley, and cracked pepper

86) Super Fresh Veggie Soup

Preparation Time: 50 minutes

Cooking Time: 0 minutes

Servings: 2

Nutrition: Calories: 255 Protein: 4 g Fat: 19.8 g Carbs: 15 g

Ingredients:

- 3 medium ripe avocados, halved, seeded, peeled, and cut to chunks
- 2 cloves fresh garlic, minced
- 2 cups low-sodium, fat-free chicken broth, divided
- ½ cucumber, peeled and chopped
- ½ cup chopped white onion
- ¼ cup finely diced carrot
- Thin avocado slices for garnish
- Paprika to sprinkle
- Freshly ground pepper to taste
- Hot red pepper sauce to taste

Directions:

- ❖ Place 6 bowls into the freezer and allow them to chill for half an hour.
- ❖ In the meantime, take out your blender and add garlic, cucumber, avocados, onion, carrot, and 1 cup broth. Blend all the ingredients together until they turn smooth.
- ❖ Add the remaining broth. Add the pepper and hot sauce to taste, if preferred.
- ❖ Blend all the ingredients again until they are smooth.
- ❖ Take out the chilled bowls and pour the blended ingredients into them.
- ❖ This time, place the bowls in the refrigerator for another 1 hour.
- ❖ When you are ready to serve, top the soup with paprika and slices of avocado.
- ❖ Serve chilled.

87) Orzo Dill Chicken Broth with Vegetables

Preparation Time: 10 minutes

Cooking Time: 40 minutes

Servings: 2

Nutrition: Calories: 248 Protein: 25 g Fat: 4 g Carbs: 23 g

Ingredients:

- 12 ounces skinless, boneless chicken breasts
- 1 tablespoon olive oil
- ½ cup chopped celery
- ½ cup chopped white onion
- 6 cups low-sodium, fat-free chicken broth
- ½ cup sliced carrot
- ½ cup orzo
- ¼ cup chopped fresh dill
- Freshly ground pepper to taste
- Lemon halves

Directions:

- ❖ Take out a large pot and place it over medium heat. Add olive oil to it and allow it to heat.
- ❖ Add celery and onion. Cook them until the onions are fragrant and the celery is soft.
- ❖ Add chicken, chicken broth, and carrot to the mixture. Add pepper to taste, if preferred.
- ❖ Increase the temperature to medium high heat and allow the broth to boil. When it starts boiling, reduce heat and allow the soup to simmer for about 20 minutes, or until the chicken is cooked.
- ❖ Take out the chicken from the pot, transfer it to a bowl and allow it to cool. Cover the pot so that the ingredients inside are simmering. When the chicken is sufficiently cool, shred the chicken into small pieces.
- ❖ Open the cover of the pot and add orzo. Increase the heat to medium high and allow the broth to boil for about 8 minutes. Make sure that the cover is back on the pot during the boiling process.
- ❖ Remove pot from heat and add dill and the shredded chicken broth.
- ❖ Squeeze lemon juice into the broth. Serve immediately.

88) Greek Lentil Soup

Preparation Time: 10 minutes

Cooking Time: 6 hours 2 minutes

Servings: 4

Nutrition: Calories 231 Fat 20.1 g Carbs 20 g Protein 4.6 g

Ingredients:

- Soup:
- 1 cup lentils
- 1 medium sweet onion, chopped
- 2 large carrots, chopped
- 2 sticks of celery, chopped
- 4 cups veggie broth
- Olive oil to sauté
- 4 tablespoons tomato sauce
- 3 cloves garlic
- 3 bay leaves
- Black pepper, to taste
- Dried oregano, to taste
- Toppings:
- Vinegar
- Lemon juice
- Hot sauce

Directions:

- ❖ In a slow cooker, add olive oil and onion.
- ❖ Sauté for 2 minutes then add the rest of the soup ingredients.
- ❖ Put on the slow cooker's lid and Cooking Time: for 6 hours on low heat.
- ❖ Serve warm with the vinegar, lemon juice, and hot sauce.

89) White Beans and Kale Soup with Artichoke and Dried Herbs

Preparation Time: 10 minutes

Cooking Time: 20 minutes

Servings: 4

Nutrition: Calories 201 Fat 8.9 g Carbs 24.7 g Protein 15.3 g

Ingredients:

- 1 (15 ouncecan artichoke hearts
- ½ bunch kale, chopped
- 2 cups vegetable broth
- 1 tablespoon dried basil
- 1 tablespoon dried oregano
- ½ teaspoon red pepper flakes
- Black pepper, to taste
- 2 (14 ouncecans roasted tomatoes, diced
- 1 (15 ouncecan white beans, drained

Directions:

- ❖ Add all ingredients to a saucepan.
- ❖ Put on the saucepan's lid and Cooking Time: for 20 minutes on a simmer.
- ❖ Serve warm.

90) Broccoli Pasta Smoked Soup

Preparation Time: 10 minutes

Cooking Time: 4 hrs. 32 minutes

Servings: 04

Nutrition: Calories 361 Fat 16.3 g Carbs 29.3 g Protein 3.3 g

Ingredients:

- 1 large bunch broccoli
- 3 cloves garlic
- 1 medium white potato
- ¼ cup carrot, chopped
- 2 cups almond milk
- 1½ cups white beans, cooked
- 1 white onion, chopped
- ¾ teaspoon black pepper
- ½ teaspoon smoky paprika
- ⅓ cup nutritional yeast
- 1 bay leaf
- 1 cup cooked pasta

Directions:

- ❖ In a slow cooker, add olive oil and onion.
- ❖ Sauté for 2 minutes then toss in the rest of the ingredients except pasta and beans.
- ❖ Put on the slow cooker's lid and Cooking Time: for 4 hours on low heat.
- ❖ Once done, add pasta and beans to the soup and mix gently.
- ❖ Cover the soup and remove it from the heat then leave it for another 30 minutes.

91) Red Potato and Broccoli Cheesy Soup

Preparation Time: 10 minutes

Cooking Time: 25 minutes

Servings: 2

Nutrition: Calories: 350 Protein: 17 g Fat: 14 g Carbs: 42 g

Ingredients:

- 2 cups escarole leaves, rinsed and drained
- 3 tablespoons all-purpose flour
- 3 cups fresh broccoli florets
- 3 scallions, sliced
- 2 cups smoked Gouda cheese, shredded and more for garnish
- 2 cups low-sodium, fat-free chicken broth
- 1 cup almond milk
- 3 medium red-gold potatoes, chopped
- 2 cloves fresh garlic, minced
- Freshly ground pepper to taste

Directions:

- ❖ Take out a large pot and place it over medium high heat. Add potatoes, garlic, and chicken broth. Bring the mixture to a boil and reduce the heat to low. Allow the mixture to simmer for a while until you notice the potatoes begin to soften
- ❖ Use a fork and mash the potatoes slightly.
- ❖ Add broccoli, milk, and scallions. Continue to heat to a simmer until broccoli turns tender and crispy.
- ❖ Bring down the heat to low and then add the Gouda cheese. Continue stirring until the sauce thickens and the cheese melts.
- ❖ Add pepper for seasoning, if preferred. Serve the soup in 4 equal portions.
- ❖ Add additional cheese and escarole as toppings.

92) Italian Grandma's Tortellini Soup

Preparation Time: 10 minutes

Cooking Time: 30 minutes

Servings: 2

Nutrition: Calories: 213 Protein: 7 g Fat: 7 g Carbs: 26 g

Ingredients:

- 32 ounces low-sodium, fat-free chicken broth
- 3 cups fresh chicken-filled tortellini
- 1 large white onion, chopped
- 4 cloves fresh garlic, chopped
- 3 celery stalks, chopped
- 1 teaspoon minced chives
- 2 14.5-ounce cans diced tomatoes, undrained
- 2 tablespoons olive oil
- 1 teaspoon dried sweet basil
- 1 cup frozen corn
- 1 teaspoon dried thyme
- 1 cup chopped carrot
- 1 cup frozen cut green beans
- 1 cup diced raw potato

Directions:

- ❖ Take out a large pot and place it over medium heat. Add garlic, onion, celery, and olive oil. Sauté until you notice the onion and garlic become fragrant and soft.
- ❖ Add potato, basil, carrot, beans, broth, thyme, corn, and chives. Increase the heat to medium high and then bring the broth to a boil.
- ❖ When it starts boiling, reduce the heat and cover the pot. Allow the mixture to simmer for about 15 minutes, or until the vegetables become tender.
- ❖ Add tortellini and tomatoes. Remove the cover and allow the soup to simmer uncovered for about 5 minutes.
- ❖ Serve hot.

93) Asian Shiitake Soup

Preparation Time: 10 minutes

Cooking Time: 3 hrs.

Servings: 04

Nutrition: Calories 210.6 Fat 10.91g Carbs 25.6g Protein 2.1g

Ingredients:

- Congee:
- 1 cup of white rice (uncooked
- 2-inch piece fresh ginger, minced
- 4 cloves garlic, minced
- 10 cups water
- 14 dried shiitake mushrooms
- Toppings:
- Green onions
- Cilantro
- Sesame seeds
- Hot sauce
- Toasted sesame oil
- Soy sauce
- Peanuts
- Chili oil
- Shelled edamame

Directions:

- ❖ Add all the ingredients to a slow cooker.
- ❖ Put on the slow cooker's lid and Cooking Time: for 3 hours on low heat.
- ❖ Once done, garnish with desired toppings.

94) Rich Oyster Soup with Toasted Bread

Preparation Time: 5 minutes

Cooking Time: 30 minutes

Servings: 2

Nutrition: Calories: 311 Protein: 23 g Fat: 11 g Carbs: 22 g

Ingredients:

- 2 pints (about 32 ounces) fresh shucked oysters, undrained
- 4 tablespoons olive oil
- 1 cup finely chopped celery
- 3 (12-ounce) cans low-fat evaporated milk
- 6 tablespoons minced shallots
- 2 pinches of cayenne pepper (add more if you like more spice)
- toasted bread squares
- Freshly ground pepper to taste

Directions:

- ❖ Start with the oysters. Drain the liquid from them in a small bowl. Set the liquid aside since we are going to use it. Place the oysters separately.
- ❖ Run the liquid through a strainer to remove any solid materials.
- ❖ Take out a large pot and place it over medium heat. Add olive oil into it. Toss in oysters, celery, and shallots.
- ❖ Allow the ingredients to simmer for about 5 minutes, or until you notice the edges of the oysters begin to curl.
- ❖ Take a separate pot (or pan) and then heat the oyster liquid and milk. When the mixture is sufficiently warm, then pour it over the oysters. Stir all the ingredients together.
- ❖ Add pepper, and cayenne pepper to taste.
- ❖ Serve soup warm with toasted bread squares as toppings or on the side.

95) Black-Eyed Pea and All Green Soup

Preparation Time: 10 minutes

Cooking Time: 5 hrs.

Servings: 4

Nutrition: Calories 197 Fat 4 g Carbs 31 g Protein 11 g

Ingredients:

- ½ cup black eyed peas
- ½ cup brown lentils
- 1 teaspoon oil
- ½ teaspoon cumin seeds
- ½ cup onions, chopped
- 5 cloves garlic, chopped
- 1-inch piece of ginger chopped
- 1 teaspoon ground coriander
- ½ teaspoon ground cumin
- ½ teaspoon turmeric
- ¼ teaspoon black pepper
- ½ teaspoon cayenne powder
- 2 tomatoes, chopped
- ½ teaspoon lemon juice
- 2 ½ cups water
- ½ cup chopped spinach
- ½ cup small chopped green beans

Directions:

- ❖ Add olive oil and cumin seeds to a slow cooker.
- ❖ Sauté for 1 minute then toss in the rest of the ingredients.
- ❖ Put on the slow cooker's lid and Cooking Time: for 5 hours on low heat.
- ❖ Once done, garnish as desired

96) Eggplant and Tomato Soup with Parmesan Cheese

Preparation Time: 10 minutes

Cooking Time: 30 minutes

Servings: 2

Nutrition: Calories: 274 Protein: 9 g Fat: 17 g Carbs: 23 g

Ingredients:

- 3 tablespoons olive oil
- 1 (14-ounce) can low-sodium tomato and basil pasta sauce
- ½ cup chopped white onion
- 2 tablespoons Italian bread crumbs
- 2 cloves fresh garlic, minced
- 2 cups low sodium, fat-free chicken broth
- ½ cup shredded reduced-fat mozzarella cheese
- 1 small eggplant, halved and sliced thinly (about 2 cups)
- 2 tablespoons freshly grated parmesan cheese for garnish

Directions:

- ❖ Preheat the oven to 500° F. We are aiming for a broiling temperature. An oven's broiling temperature is anywhere from 500° F to 550° F.
- ❖ If you feel that you want to increase the temperature, feel free to do so when you place the dish in the oven.
- ❖ Take out a nonstick pan and place it over medium heat. Add olive oil into the pan and allow it to heat. Add the eggplant and cook for about 5 minutes, stirring occasionally.
- ❖ Add garlic and onion and continue cooking until you notice the eggplant turn into a golden-brown color.
- ❖ Add broth and sauce. Increase the heat to medium high and then allow the mixture to boil.
- ❖ When it starts boiling, lower the heat to a simmer. Continue to cook until the soup thickens.
- ❖ Take out a baking tray and line it with tin foil. Use 2 oven-safe crock bowls and place them on the tray. Split the soup into equal portions and pour them into the bowls.
- ❖ Top with bread crumbs, mozzarella cheese, and a sprinkling of parmesan cheese.
- ❖ Allow the dish to broil for about 2 to 3 minutes, or until cheese has melted and turned golden.
- ❖ Serve hot.

97) Smoked Bell Pepper Mix Soup

Preparation Time: 10 minutes

Cooking Time: 4 hrs. 5 minutes

Servings: 04

Nutrition: Calories 305 Fat 11.8 g Carbs 34.6 g Protein 7 g

Ingredients:

- 1 medium onion, diced
- 2 cloves garlic, minced
- 1 green bell pepper, diced
- 1 red bell pepper, diced
- 2 carrots, peeled and diced
- 1 medium zucchini, diced
- 1 small eggplant, diced
- 1 hot banana pepper, seeded and minced
- 1 jalapeño pepper, seeded and minced
- 1 can (28 ounce diced tomatoes
- 3 cups vegetable broth
- 1½ tablespoon chili powder
- 2 teaspoons smoked paprika
- 1 tablespoon cumin
- 2 tablespoons fresh oregano, chopped
- 2 tablespoons fresh cilantro, chopped
- Black pepper to taste
- A few dashes of liquid smoke

Directions:

- ❖ In a slow cooker, add olive oil and onion.
- ❖ Sauté for 5 minutes then toss in the rest of the ingredients.
- ❖ Put on the slow cooker's lid and Cooking Time: for 4 hours on low heat.
- ❖ Once done mix well.
- ❖ Serve warm.

98) *Mexican Minestrone*

Preparation Time: 10 minutes

Cooking Time: 20 minutes

Servings: 2

Nutrition: Calories: 228 Protein: 12 g Fat: 2 g Carbs: 43 g

Ingredients:

- One 14-ounce can fiery roasted diced tomatoes, undrained
- 4 cups fresh cauliflower florets
- 1 cup frozen baby peas
- 2 teaspoons curry powder
- ½ teaspoon cumin
- 1 tablespoon finely chopped Serrano chili pepper
- 1 cup frozen corn
- cooked couscous
- 2 cloves fresh garlic, finely minced
- One 15-ounce can chickpeas, drained
- ¾ cup solid packed canned pumpkin mash
- ¾ cup water
- Freshly ground pepper to taste

Directions:

- ❖ Take a pot and place it over medium high heat. Cover it partially with water and add the cauliflower florets into it.
- ❖ Bring the water to a boil and then place the cover on the pot. Allow the florets to steam until they are tender.
- ❖ Remove the pot from the heat and drain the florets well. Cut them into small pieces and set aside.
- ❖ Take out a non-stick skillet and place it over medium heat. In a large, non-stick skillet over medium heat, add cumin and curry powder until fragrant. Add chili pepper, garlic, pumpkin, tomatoes with juices, chickpeas, and water.
- ❖ Allow the ingredients to reach a boil and then lower the heat. Let them simmer for about a minute before you add the salt and pepper to taste, if you prefer. Keep the ingredients simmering for another 15 minutes.
- ❖ Add the corn and peas and let the ingredients simmer for another 5 minutes.
- ❖ Remove from the heat and serve the soup separately with couscous or serve it over the couscous. You can also make use of brown rice instead of couscous.

99) *Green Soup With Garlic Potatoes*

Preparation Time: 10 minutes

Cooking Time: 5hrs. 5 minute

Servings: 06

Nutrition: Calories 162 Fat 4 g Carbs 17.8 g Protein 4 g

Ingredients:

- 8 ounces potatoes, diced
- 1 medium onion, chopped
- 1 large clove of garlic, chopped
- 1 teaspoon powdered mustard
- 3 cups water
- Ground cayenne pepper
- ½ cup packed fresh dill
- 10 ounces frozen spinach

Directions:

- ❖ In a low cooker, add olive oil and onion.
- ❖ Sauté for 5 minutes then toss in rest of the soup ingredients.
- ❖ Put on the slow cooker's lid and Cooking Time: for 5 hours on low heat.
- ❖ Once done, puree the soup with a hand blender.
- ❖ Serve warm.

100) *Coco Cream Zucchini Soup*

Preparation Time: 15 minutes

Cooking Time: 20 minutes

Servings: 2

Nutrition: Calories: 154 Carbs: 8.9g Fats: 8.1g Proteins: 13.4g

Ingredients:

- ½ medium onion, peeled and chopped
- 1 cup bone broth
- 1 tablespoon coconut oil
- 1½ zucchinis, cut into chunks
- ½ tablespoon nutrition al yeast
- Dash of black pepper
- ½ tablespoon parsley, chopped, for garnish
- ½ tablespoon coconut cream, for garnish

Directions:

- ❖ Melt the coconut oil in a large pan over medium heat and add onions. Sauté for about 3 minutes and add zucchinis and bone broth.
- ❖ Reduce the heat to simmer for about 15 minutes and cover the pan. Add nutrition al yeast and transfer to an immersion blender.
- ❖ Blend until smooth and season with black pepper. Top with coconut cream and parsley to serve.

Chapter 7 -   Snack Recipe

101) *Sugar Carrots with Black pepper*

Preparation Time: 10 minutes

Cooking Time: 10 minutes

Servings: 4

Nutrition: Calories 119 Fat 14 g Carbs 19 g Protein 5g

Ingredients:

- 2 cups baby carrots
- 1 tablespoon brown sugar
- ½ tablespoon vegan butter, melted
- A pinch of black pepper

Directions:

❖ Take a baking dish suitable to fit in your air fryer.

❖ Toss the leeks with butter and black pepper in the dish.

❖ Place the dish in the air fryer basket.

❖ Seal the fryer and Cooking Time: the carrots for 7 minutes at 350 degrees F on air fryer mode.

❖ Add a drizzle of lemon juice.

❖ Take a baking dish suitable to fit in your air fryer.

❖ Toss carrots with sugar, butter, salt and black pepper in the baking dish.

❖ Place the dish in the air fryer basket and seal the fryer.

❖ Cooking Time: the carrots for 10 minutes at 350 degrees F on air fryer mode.

❖ Enjoy.

102) *Fat Free Creamy Celery*

Preparation Time: 15 Minutes

Cooking Time: 20 Minutes

Servings: 3

Nutrition: Calories: 64 Carbs: 2g Fat: 6g Protein: 1g

Ingredients:

- Olive oil
- 1 clove garlic, minced
- 2 tbsp Pine nuts
- 2 tbsp dry-roasted sunflower seeds
- ¼ cup Italian cheese blend, shredded
- 8 stalks celery leaves
- 1 (8-ounce) fat-free cream cheese
- Cooking spray

Directions:

❖ Sauté garlic and pine nuts over a medium setting for the heat until the nuts are golden brown. Cut off the wide base and tops from celery.

❖ Remove two thin strips from the round side of the celery to create a flat surface.

❖ Mix Italian cheese and cream cheese in a bowl and spread into cut celery stalks.

❖ Sprinkle half of the celery pieces with sunflower seeds and a half with the pine nut mixture. Cover mixture and let stand for at least 4 hours before eating.

103) *Red Sprouts with Green Onion*

Preparation Time: 10 minutes

Cooking Time: 10 minutes

Servings: 4

Nutrition: Calories 361 Fat 16.3 g Carbs 29.3 g Protein 3.3 g

Ingredients:

- 1-pound brussels sprouts, trimmed
- ¼ cup green onions, chopped
- 6 cherry tomatoes, halved
- 1 tablespoon olive oil
- Black pepper to taste

Directions:

❖ Take a baking dish suitable to fit in your air fryer.

❖ Toss brussels sprouts with black pepper in the dish.

❖ Place this dish in the air fryer and seal the fryer.

❖ Cooking Time: the sprouts for 10 minutes at 350 degrees F on air fryer mode.

❖ Toss these sprouts with green onions, tomatoes, olive oil, and pepper in a salad bowl.

❖ Devour.

104) *Figs and Olives Spanish Tapa*

Preparation Time: 5 Minutes

Cooking Time: 0 Minutes

Servings: 1

Nutrition: Calories: 249 Carbs: 64g Fat: 1g Protein: 3g

Ingredients:

- 1 cup Dried figs
- 1 cup Kalamata olives
- ½ cup Water
- 1 tbsp Chopped fresh thyme
- 1 tbsp extra virgin olive oil
- ½ tsp Balsamic vinegar

Directions:

❖ Prepare figs in a food processor until well chopped, add water, and continue processing to form a paste.

❖ Add olives and pulse until well blended. Add thyme, vinegar, and extra virgin olive oil and pulse until very smooth. Best served with crackers of your choice.

105) *Air Fried Cheesy Asparagus*

Preparation Time: 10 minutes

Cooking Time: 8 minutes

Servings: 4

Nutrition: Calories 201 Total Fat 8.9 g Carbs 24.7 g Protein 15.3 g

Ingredients:

- 2 pounds fresh asparagus, trimmed
- ½ teaspoon oregano, dried
- 4 ounces vegan feta cheese, crumbled
- 4 garlic cloves, minced
- 2 tablespoons parsley, chopped
- ¼ teaspoon red pepper flakes
- ¼ cup olive oil
- Black pepper to the taste
- 1 teaspoon lemon zest
- 1 lemon, juiced

Directions:

- ❖ Combine lemon zest with oregano, pepper flakes, garlic and oil in a large bowl.
- ❖ Add asparagus, pepper, and cheese to the bowl.
- ❖ Toss well to coat then place the asparagus in the air fryer basket.
- ❖ Seal the fryer and Cooking Time: them for 8 minutes at 350 degrees F on Air fryer mode.
- ❖ Garnish with parsley and lemon juice.
- ❖ Enjoy warm.

106) *Crispy Potato in E.V. Olive Oil*

Preparation Time: 15 Minutes

Cooking Time: 0 Minutes

Servings: 4

Nutrition: Calories: 150 Carbs: 16g Fat: 9g Protein: 1g

Ingredients:

- 1 large Sweet potato
- 1 tbsp Extra virgin olive oil

Directions:

- ❖ 300°F preheated oven. Slice your potato into nice, thin slices that resemble fries.
- ❖ Toss the potato slices with extra virgin olive oil in a bowl. Bake for about one hour, flipping every 15 minutes until crispy and browned.

107) *Garlic Artichokes with Modena Balsamic Vinegar*

Preparation Time: 10 minutes

Cooking Time: 7 minutes

Servings: 04

Nutrition: Calories 119 Fat 14 g Carbs 19 g Protein 5g

Ingredients:

- 4 big artichokes, trimmed
- ¼ cup olive oil
- 2 garlic cloves, minced
- 2 tablespoons lemon juice
- 2 teaspoons Modena balsamic vinegar
- 1 teaspoon oregano, dried
- Black pepper to the taste

Directions:

- ❖ Season artichokes liberally with salt and pepper then rub them with half of the lemon juice and oil.
- ❖ Add the artichokes to a baking dish suitable to fit in the air fryer.
- ❖ Place the artichoke dish in the air fryer basket and seal it.
- ❖ Cooking Time: them for 7 minutes at 360 degrees F on air fryer mode.
- ❖ Whisk remaining lemon juice, and oil, vinegar, oregano, garlic and pepper in a bowl.
- ❖ Pour this mixture over the artichokes and mix them well.
- ❖ Enjoy

108) *Pita Chips with Red Hummus*

Preparation Time: 15 Minutes

Cooking Time: 20 Minutes

Servings: 4

Nutrition: Calories: 130 Carbs: 18g Fat: 5g Protein: 4g

Ingredients:

- 4 cups pita chips
- 1 (8 oz.) red pepper (roasted)
- Hummus
- 1 tsp Finely shredded lemon peel
- ¼ cup Chopped pitted Kalamata olives
- ¼ cup crumbled feta cheese
- 1 plum (Roma) tomato, seeded, chopped
- ½ cup chopped cucumber
- 1 tsp Chopped fresh oregano leaves

Directions:

- ❖ 400°F preheated oven. Arrange the pita chips on a heatproof platter and drizzle with hummus.
- ❖ Top with olives, tomato, cucumber, and cheese and bake until warmed through. Sprinkle lemon zest and oregano and enjoy while it's hot.

109) *Cherry Kebabs with Feta and Balsamic Dressing*

Preparation Time: 10 minute

Cooking Time: 6 minutes

Servings: 04

Nutrition: Calories 231 Fat 20.1 g Carbs 20 g Protein 4.6 g

Ingredients:
- 3 tablespoons balsamic vinegar
- 24 cherry tomatoes
- 2 cups vegan feta cheese, sliced
- 2 tablespoons olive oil
- 3 garlic cloves, minced
- 1 tablespoon thyme, chopped
- Black pepper to the taste
- Dressing:
- 2 tablespoons balsamic vinegar
- 4 tablespoons olive oil
- Black pepper to taste

Directions:
- ❖ In a medium bowl combine oil, garlic cloves, thyme, vinegar, and black pepper.
- ❖ Mix well then add the tomatoes and coat them liberally.
- ❖ Thread 6 tomatoes and cheese slices on each skewer alternatively.
- ❖ Place these skewers in the air fryer basket and seal it.
- ❖ Cooking Time: them for 6 minutes on air fryer mode at 360 degrees F.
- ❖ Meanwhile, whisk together the dressing ingredients.
- ❖ Place the cooked skewers on the serving plates.
- ❖ Pour the vinegar dressing over them.
- ❖ Enjoy.

110) *Kalamata Hummus Bread*

Preparation Time: 5 Minutes

Cooking Time: 0 Minutes

Servings: 3

Nutrition: Calories: 225 Carbs: 40g Fat: 5g Protein: 9g

Ingredients:
- 7 pita bread cut into 6 wedges each
- 1 (7 ounces) container plain hummus
- 1 tbsp Greek vinaigrette
- ½ cup Chopped pitted Kalamata olives

Directions:
- ❖ Spread the hummus on a serving plate— Mix vinaigrette and olives in a bowl and spoon over the hummus. Enjoy with wedges of pita bread.

111) *Veggie Cube Snack*

Preparation Time: 10 minutes

Cooking Time: 8 minutes

Servings: 4

Nutrition: Calories 361 Fat 16.3 g Carbs 29.3 g Protein 3.3 g

Ingredients:
- 1 eggplant, cubed
- 3 zucchinis, cubed
- 2 tablespoons lemon juice
- 1 teaspoon oregano, dried
- 3 tablespoons olive oil
- 1 teaspoon thyme, dried
- Black pepper to taste

Directions:
- ❖ Take a baking dish suitable to fit in your air fryer.
- ❖ Combine all ingredients in the baking dish.
- ❖ Place the eggplant dish in the air fryer basket and seal it.
- ❖ Cooking Time: them for 8 minutes at 360 degrees F on air fryer mode.
- ❖ Enjoy warm.

112) *Fresh Baked Asparagus Snack*

Preparation Time: 15 Minutes

Cooking Time: 5 Minutes

Servings: 4

Nutrition: Calories: 123 Carbs: 5g Fat: 11g Protein: 3g

Ingredients:
- 1 tbsp Extra virgin olive oil (1 tablespoon)
- Fresh Asparagus
- 1 medium lemon
- ½ tsp Freshly grated nutmeg
- ½ tsp black pepper

Directions:
- ❖ Warm the oven to 500°F. Put the asparagus on an aluminum foil and drizzle with extra virgin olive oil, and toss until well coated.
- ❖ Roast the asparagus in the oven for about five minutes; toss and continue roasting until browned. Sprinkle the roasted asparagus with nutmeg, zest, and pepper.

113) *Rosemary and Paprika Potatoes*

Preparation Time: 10 Minutes

Cooking Time: 35 Minutes

Servings: 4

Nutrition: Calories: 225 Fat: 7g Carbs: 37g Protein: 5g

Ingredients:
- 2 pounds new yellow potatoes, scrubbed and cut into wedges
- 2 tablespoons extra virgin olive oil
- 2 teaspoons fresh rosemary, chopped
- 1 teaspoon garlic powder
- 1 teaspoon sweet paprika
- ½ teaspoon freshly ground black pepper

Directions:
- ❖ Pre-heat your oven to 400 degrees Fahrenheit.
- ❖ Take a large bowl and add potatoes, olive oil, garlic, rosemary, paprika and pepper.
- ❖ Spread potatoes in single layer on baking sheet and bake for 35 minutes.
- ❖ Serve and enjoy!

114) *Air Fried Garlic Mustard Green*

Preparation Time: 10 minutes

Cooking Time: 11 minutes

Servings: 04

Nutrition: Calories 201 Fat 8.9 g Carbs 24.7 g Protein 15.3 g

Ingredients:

- 2 garlic cloves, minced
- 1 tablespoon olive oil
- ½ cup yellow onion, sliced
- 3 tablespoons vegetable stock
- ¼ teaspoon dark sesame oil
- 1-pound mustard greens, torn
- Black pepper to the taste

Directions:

- ❖ Take a baking dish suitable to fit in your air fryer.
- ❖ Add oil and place it over the medium heat and sauté onions in it for 5 minutes.
- ❖ Stir in garlic, greens, pepper, and stock.
- ❖ Mix well then place the dish in the air fryer basket.
- ❖ Seal it and Cooking Time: them for 6 minutes at 350 degrees F on air fryer mode.
- ❖ Drizzle sesame oil over the greens.
- ❖ Serve!

115) *Spicy Potato Fries*

Preparation Time: 10 Minutes

Cooking Time: 35 Minutes

Servings: 5

Nutrition: Calories 28 Fat 2.9 Fiber 0.2 Carbs 0.6 Protein 0.2

Ingredients:

- 1 teaspoon Zaatar spices
- 3 sweet potatoes
- 1 tablespoon dried dill
- 3 teaspoons sunflower oil
- ½ teaspoon paprika

Directions:

- ❖ Pour water into the crockpot. Cut the sweet potatoes into fries.
- ❖ Line the baking tray with parchment. Place the layer of the sweet potato in the tray.
- ❖ Sprinkle the vegetables with dried dill, and paprika. Then sprinkle sweet potatoes with Za'atar and mix up well with the help of the fingertips.
- ❖ Sprinkle the sweet potato fries with sunflower oil—Preheat the oven to 375F.
- ❖ Bake the sweet potato fries within 35 minutes. Stir the fries every 10 minutes.

116) *Brussels Sprouts with Vegan Parmesan*

Preparation Time: 10 minutes

Cooking Time: 8 minutes

Servings: 4

Nutrition: Calories 119 Fat 14 g Carbs 19 g Protein 5g

Ingredients:

- 1-pound brussels sprouts, washed
- 3 tablespoons vegan parmesan, grated
- Juice from 1 lemon
- 2 tablespoons vegan butter
- Black pepper to the taste

Directions:

- ❖ Spread the brussels sprouts in the air fryer basket.
- ❖ Seal it and Cooking Time: them for 8 minutes at 350 degrees F on air fryer mode.
- ❖ Place a nonstick pan over medium high heat and add butter to melt.
- ❖ Stir in pepper, lemon juice, and brussels sprouts.
- ❖ Mix well then add parmesan.
- ❖ Serve warm.

117) *Chicken SeaTime Rolls*

Preparation Time: 15 Minutes

Cooking Time: 0 Minutes

Servings: 4

Nutrition: Calories: 278 Fat: 4g Carbs: 28g Protein: 27g

Ingredients:

- 2 cups cooked chicken, chopped
- ½ English cucumbers, diced
- ½ red bell pepper, diced
- ½ cup carrot, shredded
- 1 scallion, white and green parts, chopped
- ¼ cup plain Greek yogurt
- 1 tablespoon freshly squeezed lemon juice
- ½ teaspoon fresh thyme, chopped
- Pinch of ground black pepper
- 4 multigrain tortillas

Directions:

- ❖ Take a medium bowl and mix in chicken, red bell pepper, cucumber, carrot, yogurt, scallion, lemon juice, thyme and pepper.
- ❖ Mix well.
- ❖ Spoon one quarter of chicken mix into the middle of the tortilla and fold the opposite ends of the tortilla over the filling.
- ❖ Roll the tortilla from the side to create a snug pocket.
- ❖ Repeat with the remaining ingredients and serve.
- ❖ Enjoy!

118) *Mushroom Poblano Snack with Cilantro*

Preparation Time: 10 minutes

Cooking Time: 20 minutes

Servings: 10

Nutrition: Calories 231 Fat 20 g Carbs 20.1 g Protein 4.6 g

Ingredients:

- 10 poblano peppers, tops cut off and seeds removed
- 2 teaspoons garlic, minced
- 8 ounces mushrooms, chopped
- ½ cup cilantro, chopped
- 1 white onion, chopped
- 1 tablespoon olive oil
- Black pepper to taste

Directions:

- ❖ Place a nonstick pan over medium heat and add oil.
- ❖ Stir in mushrooms and onion, sauté for 5 minutes.
- ❖ Add black pepper, cilantro and garlic.
- ❖ Stir while cooking for 2 additional minutes then take it off the heat.
- ❖ Divide this mixture in the poblano peppers and stuff them neatly.
- ❖ Place the peppers in the air fryer basket and seal it.
- ❖ Cooking Time: them for 15 minutes at 350 degrees F on air fryer mode.
- ❖ Enjoy.

119) *Juiced Ginger Bean*

Preparation Time: 5 minutes

Cooking Time: 6 minutes

Servings: 4

Nutrition: Calories: 374 Fat: 14 g Carbs: 46 g Protein: 15 g

Ingredients:

- 15.5 ounces cooked black beans
- 1 teaspoon minced garlic
- ½ of a lime, juiced
- 1 inch of ginger, grated
- 1/3 teaspoon ground black pepper
- 1 tablespoon olive oil

Directions:

- ❖ Take a frying pan, add oil and when hot, add garlic and ginger and Cooking Time: for 1 minute until fragrant.
- ❖ Then add beans, splash with some water and fry for 3 minutes until hot.
- ❖ Season beans with black pepper, drizzle with lime juice, then remove the pan from heat and mash the beans until smooth pasta comes together.
- ❖ Serve the dip with whole-grain breadsticks or vegetables.

120) *Greek Sweety Fig*

Preparation Time: 5 minutes

Cooking Time: 0 minutes

Servings: 2

Nutrition: Calories 208 Fat 3 g Carbs 39 g Protein 9 g

Ingredients:

- 6 dried figs, sliced
- 4 teaspoons honey
- 1 1/3 cups low- fat plain Greek style yogurt

Directions:

- ❖ Divide the figs into 2 bowls. Add honey and yogurt into a bowl and stir. Pour over the figs and serve.

Chapter 8 -   Dessert and Smoothie Recipes

121) _Power Banana Bars_

Preparation Time: 15 minutes

Cooking Time: 40 minutes

Servings: 16 bars

Nutrition: Calories: 145 Fat: 7.2g Protein: 3.1g Carbs: 18.9g

Ingredients:
- 2 tablespoon extra-virgin olive oil
- 2 medium ripe bananas, mashed
- ½ cup almond butter
- ½ cup maple syrup
- 1/3 cup dried cranberries
- 1½ cups old-fashioned rolled oats
- ¼ cup oat flour
- ¼ cup ground flaxseed
- ¼ teaspoon ground cloves
- ½ cup shredded coconut
- ½ teaspoon ground cinnamon
- 1 teaspoon vanilla extract

Directions:
- ❖ Preheat the oven to 400°F (205°C). Line an 8-inch square pan with parchment paper, then grease with olive oil.
- ❖ Combine the mashed bananas, almond butter, and maple syrup in a bowl. Stir to mix well. Mix in the remaining ingredients and stir to mix well until thick and sticky.
- ❖ Spread the mixture evenly on the square pan with a spatula, then bake in the preheated oven for 40 minutes or until a toothpick inserted in the center comes out clean.
- ❖ Remove them from the oven and slice into 16 bars to serve.

122) _Orange Cantaloupe Wine Smoothie_

Preparation Time: 10 minutes

Cooking Time:

Servings: 2

Nutrition: Calories 349, Fat 13.1g, Carbs 50.5g, Protein 6.5g,

Ingredients:
- 1½ cups cantaloupe, diced
- 2 Tbsp frozen orange juice concentrate
- ¼ cup white wine
- 2 ice cubes
- 1 Tbsp lemon juice
- ½ cup Mint leaves, for garnish

Directions:
- ❖ Blend all ingredients to create a smooth mixture.
- ❖ Top with mint leaves, and serve.

123) _Maple Cranberry and Quinoa Balls_

Preparation Time: 15 minutes

Cooking Time: 0 minutes

Servings: 12 balls

Nutrition: Calories: 110 Fat: 10.8g Protein: 3.1g Carbs: 4.9g

Ingredients:
- 2 tablespoons almond butter
- 2 tablespoons maple syrup
- ¾ cup cooked quinoa
- 1 tablespoon dried cranberries
- 1 tablespoon chia seeds
- ¼ cup ground almonds
- ¼ cup sesame seeds, toasted
- Zest of 1 orange
- ½ teaspoon vanilla extract

Directions:
- ❖ Line a baking sheet with parchment paper. Combine the butter and maple syrup in a bowl. Stir to mix well.
- ❖ Fold in the remaining ingredients and stir until the mixture holds together and smooth. Divide the mixture into 12 equal parts, then shape each part into a ball.
- ❖ Arrange the balls on the baking sheet, then refrigerate for at least 15 minutes. Serve chilled.

124) _Greek Cucumber Kale Smoothie_

Preparation Time: 3 minutes

Cooking Time:

Servings: 2

Nutrition: Calories 509, Fat 8.9g, Carbs 87.1g, Protein 30.6g

Ingredients:
- 1 cup Greek yogurt
- 1½ cups cubed pineapple
- 3 cups baby kale
- 1 cucumber
- 2 tbsp, hemp seeds

Directions:
- ❖ Pop everything in a blender and blitz
- ❖ Pour into glasses and serve.

125) _Dark Chilled Cherry_

Preparation Time: 15 minutes

Cooking Time: 3 minutes

Servings: 10 clusters

Nutrition: Calories: 197 Fat: 13.2g Protein: 4.1g Carbs: 17.8g

Ingredients:
- 1 cup dark chocolate (60% cocoa or higher), chopped
- 1 tablespoon coconut oil
- ½ cup dried cherries
- 1 cup roasted almonds

Directions:
- ❖ Line a baking sheet with parchment paper. Melt the chocolate and coconut oil in a saucepan for 3 minutes. Stir constantly.
- ❖ Turn off the heat and mix in the cherries and almonds. Drop the mixture on the baking sheet with a spoon. Place the sheet in the refrigerator and chill for at least 1 hour or until firm. Serve chilled.

126) *Spinach Berry Coconut Smoothie*

Preparation Time: 3 minutes

Cooking Time:

Servings: 2

Nutrition: Calories 298, Carbs 20g, Protein 4.7g

Ingredients:

- 1 cup frozen berries
- 1 cup kale or spinach
- ¾ cup coconut milk
- ½ tbsp chia seeds

Directions:

- ❖ Pop everything in a blender and blitz
- ❖ Pour into glasses and serve.

127) *Maple Cover Pears*

Preparation Time: 15 minutes

Cooking Time: 20 minutes

Servings: 4

Nutrition: Calories: 287 Fat: 3.1g Protein: 2.2g Carbs: 66.9g

Ingredients:

- 4 pears, peeled, cored, and quartered lengthwise
- 1 cup apple juice
- 1 tablespoon grated fresh ginger
- ½ cup pure maple syrup
- ¼ cup chopped hazelnuts

Directions:

- ❖ Put the pears in a pot, then pour in the apple juice. Bring to a boil over medium-high heat, then reduce the heat to medium-low. Stir constantly.
- ❖ Cover and simmer for an additional 15 minutes or until the pears are tender.
- ❖ Meanwhile, combine the ginger and maple syrup in a saucepan. Bring to a boil over medium-high heat. Stir frequently. Turn off the heat and transfer the syrup to a small bowl and let sit until ready to use.
- ❖ Transfer the pears in a large serving bowl with a slotted spoon, then top the pears with syrup. Spread the hazelnuts over the pears and serve immediately.

128) *All Colors Soy Smoothie*

Preparation Time: 5 minutes

Cooking Time:

Servings:2

Nutrition: Calories 269, Fat 12.3g, Carbs 37.6g, Protein 6.4g

Ingredients:

- ½ avocado
- 1 cup frozen blueberries
- 1 cup raw spinach
- 1 cup soy
- 1 frozen banana

Directions:

- ❖ Blend everything in a powerful blender until you have a smooth, creamy shake.
- ❖ Enjoy your healthy shake and start your
- ❖ morning on a fresh note!

129) *Italian Super Cold Granita*

Preparation Time: 15 minutes

Cooking Time: 0 minutes

Servings: 4

Nutrition: Calories: 183 Fat: 1.1g Protein: 2.2g Carbs: 45.9g

Ingredients:

- 1 pound (454 g) fresh blackberries
- 1 teaspoon chopped fresh thyme
- ¼ cup freshly squeezed lemon juice
- ½ cup raw honey
- ½ cup water

Directions:

- ❖ Put all the ingredients in a food processor, then pulse to purée. Pour the mixture through a sieve into a baking dish. Discard the seeds remain in the sieve.
- ❖ Put the baking dish in the freezer for 2 hours. Remove the dish from the refrigerator and stir to break any frozen parts.
- ❖ Return the dish back to the freezer for an hour, then stir to break any frozen parts again. Return the dish to the freezer for 4 hours until the granita is completely frozen.
- ❖ Remove it from the freezer and mash to serve.

130) *Red Banana Choco Shake*

Preparation Time: 10 minutes

Cooking Time:

Servings: 2

Nutrition: Calories 272, Fat 14.3g, Carbs 37g, Protein 6.2g

Ingredients:

- ❖ 2 frozen ripe bananas, chopped
- ❖ 1/3 cup frozen strawberries
- ❖ 2 tbsp cocoa powder
- ❖ 2 tbsp salted almond butter
- ❖ 2 cups unsweetened vanilla almond milk
- ❖ 1 dash Stevia or agave nectar
- ❖ 1/3 cup ice

Directions:

- ❖ Add all ingredients in a blender and blend until smooth.
- ❖ Take out and serve.

131) _Cheesy Cucumber on Bread_

Preparation Time: 5 minutes

Cooking Time: 0 minutes

Servings: 12

Nutrition: Calories 187 Fat 12.4g Carbs 4.5g Protein 8.2g

Ingredients:

- 1 cucumber, sliced
- 8 slices whole wheat bread
- 2 tablespoons cream cheese, soft
- 1 tablespoon chives, chopped
- ¼ cup avocado, peeled, pitted and mashed
- 1 teaspoon mustard
- Black pepper to the taste

Directions:

- ❖ Spread the mashed avocado on each bread slice, also spread the rest of the ingredients except the cucumber slices.
- ❖ Divide the cucumber slices on the bread slices, cut each slice in thirds, arrange on a platter and serve as an appetizer.

132) _Kale with Berries Mix Smoothie_

Preparation Time: 5 minutes

Cooking Time:

Servings: 2

Nutrition: Calories 164, Total Fat 2g, Carbs 34.2g, Protein 4.1g

Ingredients:

- ❖ 1 medium ripe banana, peeled and sliced
- ❖ ½ cup frozen mixed berries
- ❖ 1 tbsp hulled hemp seeds
- ❖ 2 cups frozen or fresh kale
- ❖ 2/3 cup 100% pomegranate juice
- ❖ 2¼ cups filtered water

Directions:

- ❖ Add all ingredients in a blender and blend until smooth.
- ❖ Take out and serve.

133) _Zaatar Kalamata Greek Dip_

Preparation Time: 10 minutes

Cooking Time: 0 minutes

Servings: 6

Nutrition: Calories 294 Fat 18g Carbs 2g Protein 10g

Ingredients:

- 2 cups Greek yogurt
- 2 tablespoons pistachios, toasted and chopped
- A pinch of white pepper
- 2 tablespoons mint, chopped
- 1 tablespoon kalamata olives, pitted and chopped
- ¼ cup zaatar spice
- ¼ cup pomegranate seeds
- 1/3 cup olive oil

Directions:

- ❖ Mix the yogurt with the pistachios and the rest of the ingredients, whisk well, divide into small cups and serve with pita chips on the side.

134) _Raspberry Agave Juice_

Preparation Time: 5 minutes

Cooking Time:

Servings: 2

Nutrition: Calories 227, Fat 4g, Carbs 47.8g, Protein 0.9g

Ingredients:

- ❖ 1 cup water
- ❖ 1 cup fresh or frozen raspberries
- ❖ 1 large frozen banana
- ❖ 2 tbsp fresh juice, lime
- ❖ 1 tsp oil, coconut
- ❖ 1 tsp agave

Directions:

- ❖ In a blender put all ingredients and blend until smooth.
- ❖ Take out and serve

135) _Nectarines and Figs Crumble_

Preparation Time: 15 minutes

Cooking Time: 15 minutes

Servings: 6

Nutrition: Calories: 336 Fat: 18.8g Protein: 6.3g Carbs: 41.9g

Ingredients:

- Topping:
- ¼ cup coarsely chopped hazelnuts
- 1 cup coarsely chopped walnuts
- 1 teaspoon ground cinnamon
- 1 tablespoon melted coconut oil
- Filling:
- 6 fresh figs, quartered
- 2 nectarines, pitted and sliced
- 1 cup fresh blueberries
- 2 teaspoons lemon zest
- ½ cup raw honey
- 1 teaspoon vanilla extract

Directions:

- ❖ Combine the ingredients for the topping in a bowl. Stir to mix well. Set aside until ready to use.
- ❖ Preheat the oven to 375°F (190°C). Combine the ingredients for the fillings in a bowl. Stir to mix well. Divide the filling in six ramekins, then divide and top with nut topping.
- ❖ Bake in the preheated oven for 15 minutes or until the topping is lightly browned and the filling is frothy. Serve immediately.

136) *Plant-Based Banana and Spinach Smoothie*

Preparation Time: 5 minutes

Cooking Time:

Servings: 1

Nutrition: Calories 364, Fat 4.8g, Carbs 78g, Protein 9.6g

Ingredients:

- 1 cup coconut water
- ¾ cup plant-based milk
- ¼ tsp vanilla extract
- 1 heaping cup loosely packed spinach
- 2-3 cups frozen bananas, sliced

Directions:

- ❖ Blend everything until smooth and serve.

137) *Wrong After Eight Sorbet*

Preparation Time: 4 hours & 5 minutes

Cooking Time: 0 minutes

Servings: 1

Nutrition: Calories: 213 Fat: 9.8g Protein: 3.1g Carbs: 2.9g

Ingredients:

- 1 frozen banana
- 1 tablespoon almond butter
- 2 tablespoons minced fresh mint
- 2 to 3 tablespoons dark chocolate chips (60% cocoa or higher)
- 2 to 3 tablespoons goji (optional)

Directions:

- ❖ Put the banana, butter, and mint in a food processor. Pulse to purée until creamy and smooth. Add the chocolate and goji, then pulse for several more times to combine well.
- ❖ Pour the mixture in a bowl or a ramekin, then freeze for at least 4 hours before serving chilled.

138) *Exotic Mix Crushed Smoothie*

Preparation Time: 5 minutes

Cooking Time:

Servings: 2

Nutrition: Calories 269, Fat 12.3g, Carbs 37.6g, Protein 6.4g,

Ingredients:

- 1 cup orange slices
- 1 cup mango chunks
- 1 cup strawberries, chopped
- 1 cup coconut water
- Pinch freshly grated ginger
- 1-2 cups crushed ice

Directions:

- ❖ Place everything in a blender, blend, and serve.

139) *Cinnamon Maple Carrot Cake*

Preparation Time: 15 minutes

Cooking Time: 45 minutes

Servings: 12

Nutrition: Calories: 255 Fat: 19.2g Protein: 5.1g Carbs: 12.8g

Ingredients:

- ½ cup coconut oil, at room temperature, plus more for greasing the baking dish
- 2 teaspoons pure vanilla extract
- ¼ cup pure maple syrup
- 6 eggs
- ½ cup coconut flour
- 1 teaspoon baking powder
- 1 teaspoon baking soda
- ½ teaspoon ground nutmeg
- 1 teaspoon ground cinnamon
- ½ cup chopped pecans
- 3 cups finely grated carrots

Directions:

- ❖ Preheat the oven to 350°F (180°C). Grease a 13-by-9-inch baking dish with coconut oil. Combine the vanilla extract, maple syrup, and ½ cup of coconut oil in a large bowl. Stir to mix well.
- ❖ Break the eggs in the bowl and whisk to combine well. Set aside. Combine the coconut flour, baking powder, baking soda, nutmeg, and cinnamon in a separate bowl. Stir to mix well.
- ❖ Make a well in the center of the flour mixture, then pour the egg mixture into the well. Stir to combine well.
- ❖ Add the pecans and carrots to the bowl and toss to mix well. Pour the mixture in the single layer on the baking dish.
- ❖ Bake in the preheated oven for 45 minutes or until puffed and the cake spring back when lightly press with your fingers.
- ❖ Remove the cake from the oven. Allow to cool for at least 15 minutes, then serve.

140) *Halloween Banana Smoothie*

Preparation Time: 5 minutes

Cooking Time:

Servings: 2

Nutrition: Calories 272, Fat 5.6g, Carbs 51.9g, Protein 8.2g

Ingredients:

- 1 cup unsweetened non-dairy milk
- 2 medium bananas, peeled and cut into quarters and frozen
- 2 medjool dates, pitted
- 1 cup pumpkin puree, canned or fresh
- 2 cups ice cubes
- ¼ tsp cinnamon
- 2 tbsp ground flaxseeds

Directions:

- ❖ Blend all ingredients in a blender and serve.

Chapter 9 - Easy Dr. Cole's Diet Plan – On a Budget

Day 1

1) Complete Cheesy Breakfast Egg | Calories 337

23) Delicious Fruity Pasta | Calories 329

64) Simple Chicken Bell Pepper | Calories 254

42) Pea Shoot Radish Salad | Calories 158

122) Orange Cantaloupe Wine Smoothie | Calories 349

Total Calories: 1427

Day 2

4) Superfood Bars with Apple Sauce | Calories 230

28) Sicilian Linguine with Mushroom Mix | Calories 331

67) Creamy Kale Broccoli with Parmesan Cheese | Calories 193

44) Baby Potato Salad with Apple Mustard Dressing | Calories 197

124) Greek Cucumber Kale Smoothie | Calories 509

Total Calories: 1460

Day 3

9) Orange Coco Shake | Calories 335

35) Pasta "Mari e Monti" | Calories 346

69) Baked Bell Peppers with Yogurt Topping | Calories 251

46) Exotic Summer Salad | Calories 305

134) Raspberry Agave Juice | Calories 227

Total Calories: 1464

Day 4

10) Sweety Avena Fruit Muffins with Walnuts | Calories 351

39) Maple Veggie Macaroni Casserole | Calories 349

71) Veggie Bacon and Tofu Rolls | Calories 260

49) Green and Lentil Cauli Salad | Calories 212

133) Zaatar Kalamata Greek Dip | Calories 294

Total Calories: 1466

Day 5

20) Berries Mix Mug Bread | Calories 165

37) Lettuce Rolls with Beans and Hummus | Calories 211

76) Crispistachio Whitefish | Calories 185

53) Broccoli and Coco Chickpea Salad with Garlic Sauce | Calories 231

135) Nectarines and Figs Crumble | Calories 336

Total Calories: 1128

Day 6

17) Baked Seed Mix Loaf | Calories 172

29) Tomato Pasta with Parmesan Cheese | Calories 265

79) Splash Beans and Potatoes with Tamari Sauce | Calories 232

55) Red Bell Fennel Salad with Tahini | Calories 205

136) Plant-Based Banana and Spinach Smoothie | Calories 364

Total Calories: 1238

Day 7

12) Green Banana Shake with Vanilla | Calories 298

25) Italian Pappardelle with Jumbo Shrimp | Calories 474

80) Sliced Cuttlefish in Robola Wine | Calories 308

59) Bulgur Mixture with Fresh Mint | Calories 271

121) Power Banana Bars | Calories 145

Total Calories: 1496

Chapter 10 - Conclusion

I hope this book of recipes will be useful to you in the long term, I remind you that the DASH diet is a diet proven by specialists from various medical disciplines, it is not just a fad or for aesthetic reasons, it will really make a difference in your life and your health.

The best medicine for our body is to take care of our diet, and if in addition to taking care of our health we can show off a better figure is the perfect deal.

Keep in mind that the portions that I include in each recipe must be careful so that the diet works properly and you get the most out of all the benefits it offers.

As a final tip, I suggest you write in your diary or in a notebook a note about how you feel before starting the diet, how you see your body, write down your weight, if you feel swollen or if you have heaviness, have any difficulty, in short your feelings in general, keep your notes and when you have at least two or three weeks of following this diet review it again and you will discover the changes that are already beginning to occur.

Much success and welcome to a healthier and happier life.

CPSIA information can be obtained
at www.ICGtesting.com
Printed in the USA
BVHW010656010721
610723BV00017B/1531